# ENTERiNG
# PRIVATE PRACTICE

*A Handbook for Psychiatrists*

# ENTERING PRIVATE PRACTICE
## A Handbook for Psychiatrists

Edited by

*Jeremy A. Lazarus, M.D.*

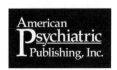

Washington, DC
London, England

**Note:** Books published by American Psychiatric Publishing, Inc., represent the views and opinions of the individual authors and do not necessarily represent the policies and opinions of APPI or the American Psychiatric Association.

Manufactured in the United States of America on acid-free paper
09   08   07   06   05     5   4   3   2   1

First Edition

Typeset in Janson Text and Bailey Sans ITC.

American Psychiatric Publishing, Inc.
1000 Wilson Boulevard
Arlington, VA 22209-3901
www.appi.org

**Library of Congress Cataloging-in-Publication Data**
Entering private practice : a handbook for psychiatrists / [edited] by Jeremy A. Lazarus.-- 1st ed.
    p. ; cm.
  Includes bibliographical references and index.
  ISBN 1-58562-141-2 (pbk. : alk. paper)
1. Psychiatry--Practice--United States.
  [DNLM: 1. Private Practice--organization & administration. 2. Psychiatry--methods. 3. Practice Management. WM 30 E61 2005] I. Lazarus, Jeremy A.

  RC465.6.E55 2005
  616.89'0068--dc22

                                                    2005008200

**British Library Cataloguing in Publication Data**
A CIP record is available from the British Library.

# CONTENTS

# CONTRIBUTORS

**Michael I. Bennett, M.D.**
Supervisory Staff, Massachusetts Mental Health Center, and Medical Director, Mental Health Case Management, Chestnut Hill, Massachusetts

**Roger G. Bonds, M.B.A., F.M.S.D., C.M.S.R.**
Chief Executive Officer, American Academy of Medical Management, Roswell, Georgia

**Marcia L. Brauchler, M.P.H., CPHQ, CPC**
President, Physicians' Ally, Inc., Highlands Ranch, Colorado

**Steven Cole, M.D.**
Professor of Clinical Psychiatry and Head, Division of Medical and Geriatric Psychiatry, S.U.N.Y. Stony Brook Health Sciences Center, Stony Brook, New York

**Jonathan M. Kersun, M.D.**
Private Practice, Swarthmore, Pennsylvania

**Jeremy A. Lazarus, M.D.**
Clinical Professor of Psychiatry, University of Colorado Health Sciences Center, Denver, Colorado

**John Luo, M.D.**
Assistant Clinical Professor of Psychiatry, UCLA Neuropsychiatric Institute and Hospital, Los Angeles, California

**Edward K. Silberman, M.D.**
Vice-Chair for Adult Services (medical school appointment pending), Department of Psychiatry, Tufts-New England Medical Center, Boston, Massachusetts

**Anne Marie "Nancy" Wheeler, J.D.**
Attorney in Private Practice; Coordinator, American Psychiatric Association Legal Consultation Plan; Affiliate Faculty, Loyola College in Maryland, Graduate Pastoral Counseling Program, Columbia, Maryland

# 1

# INTRODUCTION

*Jeremy A. Lazarus, M.D.*

For the psychiatrist who is recently trained or who is planning a career change, the prospect of entering private practice is at the same time very exciting and fraught with questions and concerns. This book was conceived after the editor's many years of organizing seminars for psychiatric residents who were trying to make career decisions. Although some residencies offer limited guidance or mentoring on entering private practice, there has been no comprehensive curricular approach—and, indeed, there is already too much to learn about the art and science of psychiatry to spend significant educational time in this area. What most psychiatrists want is practical advice from those who have experience and are experts in specialized areas. Although no one book can contain all of the information that will help in setting out on a career in private practice, this book will give the reader a substantial head start. It will also provide help in avoiding the pitfalls that have been experienced by many. For this purpose, I sought to bring together experts in marketing, job searching, buying insurance, communicating with primary care physicians, setting up a private office, using technology in the office, and dealing with legal and ethical issues. It is also crucial for the reader to ask the advice of trusted friends, colleagues, teachers, and family in arriving at the best practice situation. Don't assume you know how things will go in a particular practice setting without doing your homework. If you do your homework and follow good advice, you will get the most out of your practice.

The first critical question to ask oneself is: Does private practice offer me the type of work and living situation that will make my professional and personal life fulfilling? From over 30 years' experience in private practice,

1

and having talked with psychiatrists around the country, I think it's fair to say that there is no other place where one can experience the unencumbered joy of treating the individual patient over a short time or over decades. There is no other situation where you can be free to practice in the style and with the theoretical and scientific background that are most consistent with your training. There is no other way that you can be the sole master of your professional fate and accept both the responsibilities and the risks. But to reflect more systematically on this question, I offer the following discussion of advantages and disadvantages of private practice and then briefly discuss other activities you can be involved in to enrich your professional and personal life.

## ∎ ADVANTAGES OF THE PRIVATE PRACTICE OF PSYCHIATRY

Private practice offers many advantages:

- Autonomy
- Choice of clinical work
- Choice of range of clinical work
- Choice of area in which to live and work
- Range of income
- Flexibility

Let me discuss each of these in more detail.

### Autonomy

Being one's own boss and having the freedom to make all of one's choices as a professional are deeply held values for many, and they are most fully expressed in private practice. You can choose whom to serve, where to serve them, how much to work, where to work, with whom to work, and how much income to seek. In addition, there is the emotional and psychological sense of freedom that comes with running and owning a professional practice and business and making decisions according to your own wishes.

### Choice of Clinical Work

Although there may be limitations on the full expression of your choice of the type of patient to see when starting out in practice, over the course of time you can aim to work with the types of patients whom you feel you serve best and who are of the most interest to you professionally. You can determine whether you prefer primarily psychotherapy, psychopharmacology, psychotherapy plus psychopharmacology, individual or couples therapy, group therapy, or other modalities of therapy/treatment in which you are most expert.

## Choice of Range of Clinical Work

You can choose a fee-for-service or third-party reimbursement practice or a combination. Many psychiatrists mix treatment of full-paying patients with insurance, managed care, or preferred provider organization (PPO) practices. Through managed care or PPO practices, you may be able to request patients with a particular diagnosis or with problems that you have a particular expertise in treating.

You can also choose whether you want to work by yourself or in collaboration with other psychiatrists, physicians, or mental health professionals. I will cover this aspect in more detail in the chapter on types of private practice (Chapter 3 of this volume), but it is important to recognize the wide variety of clinical practice opportunities available.

## Choice of Area in Which to Live and Work

Although it may seem obvious, if you are entering a private practice, you have the ability to choose the state you wish to live in, an urban or rural practice, whether you want to live near to or farther from your work, and other lifestyle options that will make your personal life a gratifying one. Some psychiatrists choose to work in an urban setting and live in the suburbs or in a rural area; others do the opposite. Some psychiatrists work in multiple settings, dividing their time between an urban practice and a commuting rural or suburban practice. Ultimately, the choice of where to practice and where to live will be determined by your interests both professionally and personally.

## Range of Income

The range of income that one can expect in private practice is dependent on a host of variables. These include whether you draw from a full-fee-paying population or receive reimbursement from insurance or other third-party payers, the number of hours you work per week, and the number of patients you see per hour. With some upper limit on the number of hours you work per week, the principal way you can reasonably expect to increase your income is by doing types of work that may pay more, such as forensic, consultation, or other administrative work. It is also possible to increase income by using a physician extender model, employing other mental health professionals.

Because most psychiatrists do virtually no procedures and have no other in-office means of increasing income, we are limited to our cognitive abilities and time. Nevertheless, a decent income can be achieved with a reasonable work week. Although there are no guarantees, finding the right practice niche will usually include an assessment of future income. If you happen to be purchasing another psychiatrist's practice, additional assessment with good consultants can help you estimate your potential income. Income ranges in various parts of the country are available through both the American Psychiatric Association (APA) and the American Medical Association (AMA). APA and AMA are also good resources for other practice management information. They can be accessed on the Web at http://www.psych.org for APA and http://www.ama-assn.org for AMA. There is also valid evidence that practicing in a group may provide a higher level of income than practicing solo.

## Flexibility

As your own boss, you can decide on which days, weeks, hours, and places to work. You can work in an office part- or full-time, work in another setting part-time, volunteer at a university or clinic, volunteer for psychiatric society or medical society meetings, and take part in other activities either professionally or personally, during the work day or in the evenings. The bottom line is that your hours are yours to decide on and you can mix your professional activities with your personal activities as you wish. You have the maximum ability to plan your day and your week in a private practice setting.

Of course, in a private practice you may have increased responsibilities to patients that you may not be able to share with others. However, even in private practice, you should be able to arrange call sharing (if you wish) with other psychiatrists for evenings, weekends, or vacations. In my own practice, I have had a group of five to seven psychiatrists take evening and weekend calls without problems over the past 30 years.

## ■ DISADVANTAGES OF PSYCHIATRIC PRIVATE PRACTICE

Having gone over some of the advantages of private practice, let's now look at some of the potential disadvantages:

- Limitations on professional work
- Full responsibility for patients and business
- Uncertainty of income and benefits
- Less frequent interactions with colleagues

Let's take a look at each of these.

## Limitations on Professional Work

Let's face it: If you want to do full-time teaching, research, administration, supervision, public sector work, writing, or other scholarly work, then private practice is probably not for you. Although there are numerous opportunities to do all of these part-time, if your heart is in one of them, you probably won't be fulfilled in private practice. On the other hand, one of the advantages of private practice is that while engaged in it you can still do these other things part-time. I myself have been able to continue an active private practice, teach residents, volunteer for a free clinic, write, and be actively involved in organized psychiatry and medicine. Of course, I haven't been able to do all of these things all of the time or with full commitment to each, but you can choose your hours and the timing of your involvement.

In addition, it may be possible in another treatment setting, such as an academic center or a public or other clinic, to treat a specific type of patient that you might not be able to see in a private practice. Being able to draw from a larger volume of patients in these settings may be an advantage over private practice.

Only you can decide what will give you the most professional satisfaction—and if patient care as a primary goal is not your desire, then private practice is probably not the best way to go with your career.

## Full Responsibility for Patients and Business

Although you can always find other psychiatrists to share coverage for you, in general a private practice means that you respond to patient calls either personally or through office staff. You take full responsibility for your patients, and you either prosper or perish based on your professional and interpersonal abilities. Also, you take full responsibility for running the business aspects of your practice. Although you can get appropriate professionals and staff to help you, ultimately you are the captain of your ship and it sails or sinks under your command. In other settings, you may be able to rely on others to assist with the patient care aspects of practice as well as the business activities. You may be involved in an advisory capacity, but the business aspects are often out of your hands. This may or may not be appealing to you. Some of us really enjoy the business parts of practice, and others of us want to keep a good distance from those activities.

## Uncertainty of Income and Benefits

No matter what you project or what you are told, you can never be absolutely assured of a particular income in a private practice. Unlike a salaried position, where you can count on a certain monthly amount accompanied by various benefits, a private practice may not have a reliable cash flow that you can count on from month to month. This is especially true at the start, when you are still building up your practice and it is unlikely that your hours will be entirely taken. The benefits that are available to you in a salaried position may also be better than what you can arrange for in a private practice. Large institutions or clinics can often negotiate for better and less costly health benefits and may also be able to provide you retirement, disability, and other insurance benefits either at better rates or as part of an overall compensation package. On the other hand, as a private practitioner, you may wish to have a broader array of benefits available—at your choice rather than your employer's.

## Less Frequent Interactions With Colleagues

Depending on the type of private practice you envision, you may find yourself less connected with others in the practice setting than you were either in your residency or in an employed role. This can always be offset by practice arrangements, which I discuss in Chapter 3 of this volume, but it is fairly clear that if you are a solo practitioner, you may find yourself alone during a good part of your professional day. If you thrive on teamwork, collaboration in patient care, and time to have stimulating intellectual discussions about the science and art of psychiatry, then—unless you can find the right part-time mix to provide those opportunities—you may find private practice unfulfilling. If those types of experiences are important to you, but you don't wish them to occupy you full-time, then you can mix those activities with private practice.

## ▐ OTHER CONSIDERATIONS

Now that we have taken a look at some of the advantages and disadvantages of private practice, let's look at some of the possibilities in your professional and personal life that will enrich your private practice experience.

Although seeing patients is the primary focus of a private practice, this doesn't preclude your involvement in a wide variety of professional opportunities. You can volunteer to supervise or teach residents or medical students and be a part of the clinical faculty at a university medical center. You can volunteer to do pro bono work in clinics for the uninsured or in other community clinics. Some psychiatrists volunteer to be on the state board of medical examiners or provide services to the impaired-physician program. There are opportunities to be on committees on hospital medical staffs or in your APA district branch. You can also join your county and state medical society and volunteer for committees there. All of these provide you with opportunities to meet other psychiatrists and physicians, stay active professionally in your community, and offer possible leadership advancement opportunities. Don't expect to start at the top of the food chain in any of these settings, but time and good work will eventually pay off with even more gratifying experiences. These volunteer roles may also improve your referrals and stature in the community as well as being gratifying on their own. Contact your APA district branch and the state or country medical society, as well as the AMA, to find out what you can do to help in organized psychiatry and medicine.

If you are inclined to write, publish, or do research, private practice will limit you only in terms of time available. Some of the most interesting publications come from psychiatrists who can write about their patient experiences in real-world settings as opposed to carefully controlled studies. Research opportunities abound as companies look for broad patient groups, including groups in private settings, with which to do appropriate studies. These studies may provide interesting scientific updates and offer you the opportunity to be a part of well-designed research protocols. They also will usually provide appropriate reimbursement for your patient care so as not to significantly affect your income.

As you consider the proper balance between your professional life and your personal life, make sure that you love what you're doing in your work. That's the best advice possible if you want to have a gratifying professional life. However, also make sure that you have time for your family, friends, and significant others. Take care of yourself physically and psychologically. Do all of the things that you would advise your patients to do to stay healthy through proper diet, exercise, and attention to taking care of stress in your life. While all of these suggestions are common sense, it's important to recognize that your success in a private practice will also depend on your success in and appreciation for your personal life. If you have personal or psychological problems, don't hesitate to get treatment. Make sure that you have colleagues to talk to about difficult patients, practice concerns, and issues in your personal life that are affecting you. With these safeguards, outlets, and attention to personal concerns, you can maximize your ability to have a gratifying private practice.

## ▮ CONCLUSION

In the chapters that follow, you'll first learn in the chapter by Roger Bonds how to find a job in private practice. The multiple practice opportunities and their advantages and disadvantages are covered in my chapter on the many types of private practice. Next, Drs. Kersun and Silberman tell you how to set up a private practice office. Then you'll learn from Marcia Brauchler how to market your practice. Learning the ins and outs of insurance billing and relationships is the subject of Dr. Bennett's chapter. Dr. Luo outlines computer resources that can assist you in private practice. Knowing how to relate to primary care physicians is the focus of Dr. Cole's chapter, and you'll learn some of the legal pitfalls to look out for in Nancy Wheeler's chapter. In the final chapter, I'll discuss some common ethical problems and how to avoid or deal with them.

You can make your own list of advantages and disadvantages of private practice and see how you come out in the balance. Sometimes starting a private practice can be anxiety producing, but if it's your passion to work in a private practice setting, you will succeed.

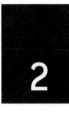

# 2 FINDING THE BEST POSITION FOR YOUR MEDICAL CAREER— AND YOUR PEACE OF MIND

*Roger G. Bonds, M.B.A., F.M.S.D., C.M.S.R.*

Each year we see thousands of graduating residents and fellows taking their first jobs as practicing physicians. Most go into private practice; others pursue careers in academia, research, and other rewarding areas. Every young physician is excited about taking the next step in a promising medical career.

Although you will certainly have a gainful position as a psychiatrist, you will want not only to have a job, but also have a career that is suited for you personally and professionally in the location and community that are best for you.

However, our research at The National Institute of Physician Career Development now shows that the average graduating physician keeps his or her first job for only 2.4 years (Bonds 2004). Because of this, many medical organizations prefer not to hire a new graduate. They want someone who has already made the first career move. But why is it that the brightest, best-educated professionals in the wealthiest nation on earth prepare years for a career only to find that the first position lasts such short a time? Let's examine the reasons.

# ■  WHY THE FIRST POSITION MAY NOT BE A GOOD FIT

## Lack of Planning

Did you know that research (Bonds 2004) shows that most graduating physicians literally spend more time planning their first vacations after graduation than they do planning their careers? For the vacation, they make phone calls, search on the Internet, discuss options with colleagues, order brochures, and have repeated conversations with their spouse or significant other. But for their careers, they generally discuss options with colleagues (the process known as networking) and then throw away most letters and brochures that are mailed to them. Most never make phone calls to inquire about advertised positions or conduct significant research on the Internet. In the end, most young doctors take the position that falls into line the easiest for them.

## Poor Follow-through

Many newly practicing physicians also make the wrong career move by making a decision that goes against what they originally wanted. For example, the physician and spouse thought they would like to live in the Midwest, where they have been living for the last few years. However, an offer of $20,000 more comes along and they jump at the chance to go to Phoenix, a place they have never visited.

## Changing Priorities

Once the newly graduated physician is in the new position and settled in, we normally see a rapid maturation, professionally and personally. The young doctor develops much more self-confidence in her clinical skills, as well as in the day-to-day operations of the practice. If she travels to different locations, she establishes a workable routine. If she is building referral relationships with physicians and other providers, she gains confidence. As she bills the insurance companies, she realizes what really can and cannot be done to have her services paid fully and faster. In time, she understands that she can confidently take these skills almost anywhere. The result of all this is a young doctor who is now at a very different level professionally. Although the partners or employers want this maturation, the young physician at this point often sees new horizons and moves on.

On the personal side, we see a similar maturation. This is a pivotal time in the young doctor's life, with a new lifestyle and new personal needs. The single greatest determinant is having children and wanting to be closer to the extended family. Also, research (Bonds 2004) shows that for the second job, a physician typically lives within 500 miles of wherever she or her spouse calls home. (Home is defined as where the person grew up or where his or her parents or other family members are now.)

## Inaccurate Expectations

Matching expectations is always difficult, whether dealing with a patient, spouse, or partner. In the case of the first job expectations, it is a difficult challenge for each young physician to ask enough questions (and receive adequate responses) to develop a realistic view of the new position. It is very common for a newly practicing physician to walk into a new position with a view of the job that differs dramatically from what the job actually entails. The same is true for the employers' or partners' expectations of the new employee. Each party expects something different. Problem areas can include hours or call coverage, pay scale, office space or location, support staff, partnership track, and innumerable other possibilities. Although the problem resides with both parties, the fact is that young physicians often leave because the position simply was not what they expected.

## Changing Relationships and Practice

When a practice or other organization brings in a young physician, the organization is by definition in a dynamic setting. That is, they are changing and evolving, which is why they signed the new doctor. Ideally this will better the organization, but often the dynamics do not work for the best. Perhaps a managed care contract is lost. If the practice cannot support its increased number of providers, it probably will cut the last one hired ("last in, first out"). Additionally, the young physician should realize that professional and personal relationships change. The practice or department members whom you adored at the outset may not be so likeable after you have been with them for a couple of years. Stress and financial problems often strain these relationships, and the grass can then seem a lot greener on the other side.

## ▌ FINDING THE RIGHT POSITION

### Career Choice Priorities

Now let's examine what motivates graduating physicians to choose that first position. Of course, money is extremely important. Young physicians are highly motivated to "catch up with the Joneses" and acquire large and small belongings such as a house, cars, clothes, and much more.

However, most say that hours worked are far more important, so they are willing to make a deal for less money if they can work fewer hours. But that is usually wishful thinking. Newly graduated physicians quickly learn that to earn a substantial income, as physicians normally do, they have to work just as hard as their older colleagues, whether in private practice or academia. The most significant exception to this pattern is the young female physician who takes a strictly hourly or part-time position so that she can spend time with her children.

Geography is also a major determinant. Young physicians tend to move first to a locale where they think they would enjoy living. For example, if you enjoyed vacationing in Florida, you might take a position there or in the next state, even though you and your spouse are from Chicago. Although this might be your best decision in the short run, as you will learn in the rest of this chapter, you can greatly reduce your newfound risk if you don't buy a house there right away and don't overspend. Then, if you beat the odds and decide to live there long-term, you will know exactly where you want to live and will have the money to buy or build a wonderful home.

Employment with a guaranteed income and benefits is also a priority. Young physicians want the security of a regular paycheck. Of course, most academic positions are defined as employment. The salary may be lower compared with the income from a private practice, but the benefits are usually much more robust. This security is a key reason so many young doctors desire academia.

For private practice, the position may be contracted or solo, partnership or employment. In each case, the base pay could be small or quite large. A productivity bonus may or may not apply, and benefits may be very good or nonexistent. A solo practice may have an income subsidy from a hospital, or it may have no subsidy and therefore no income for the first weeks or months.

To clarify definitions: *Contracted* means the physician is self-employed and contracted to work with the practice. The pay could be a set amount or could be based solely on production. *Solo* practice is defined as the physician's being on his own ("self-employed"). *Partnership* is when the physician is actually an owner of the practice, but this is usually not an option at first unless it is a new practice in which all the new physicians are made partners. *Employment* means the physician is literally an employee of the practice, which is the preferred model for most young physicians. A partnership option may then be available after 2 to 3 years.

It should be noted that going solo for the first position out of training is a common option, although sometimes a difficult one. Many newly practicing psychiatrists who choose this option have outside assistance to set up the practice. For example, hospitals often set up new practices. During the first years, the hospital may provide subsidized office space, telephone, furniture, office supplies, computer, and perhaps a shared receptionist and billing coordinator. There are medical management companies and medical office buildings that offer the same services, but they do not subsidize the services provided. Their business is to lease office space and provide associated practice services.

## No Need to Learn the Hard Way

Newly graduated physicians often do not have the experience or have not been taught some of the lessons that older physicians have learned the hard way.

First, it is imperative when evaluating a career opportunity that the doctor consider the job's total remuneration. This includes a set dollar amount for the base pay, bonus or productivity pay, and benefits. It is as simple as listing each item with a specific or estimated dollar amount and adding up the total. Unfortunately, thousands of young physicians make career decisions each year by considering only the base pay or salary. Here is an example. For simplicity, consider all the other factors of these three practices to be equal.

The graduating resident and spouse are from the upper Midwest and are now located in Chicago. There is a practice opportunity in Milwaukee, Wisconsin, offering a base of $100,000; a practice in St. Paul, Minnesota, offering $95,000; and a practice in rural Illinois offering $80,000. At first glance, most young psychiatrists are much more interested in the higher-paying practices and probably will not consider the Illinois practice. But on further examination, we find that the Wisconsin and Minnesota practices offer no bonus and the benefits include only health insurance and three weeks' vacation. However, the Illinois offer is actually a base of $80,000, with a realistic productivity bonus of $20,000, plus benefits that include health insurance, 3 weeks' vacation, 2 weeks' sick time, paid holidays, short-term disability insurance, long-term disability insurance, life insurance, dental insurance, vision insurance, $3,000 continuing medical education, and a retirement plan that contributes $15,000 per year. The total package is well over $125,000 annually. Additionally, the cost of living is significantly less in rural Illinois, resulting in a further enhanced income level for the physician.

The next major mistake that we see young doctors make is buying a home for their first career move after training. Quite simply, it usually takes several years to break even on a home if you must resell it. If you fall within the normal range and thus stay in the position for only 2.4 years, then you will probably lose thousands of dollars. Adding these dollars to the thousands you will spend on furnishing the home, plus insurance, upkeep, maid service, yard service, and so on, it all totals up to a major loss at a time when the young physician probably already has tremendous debts.

An exception to this rule may be if you are moving back to your home town where you have much more confidence in staying long-term. Another is if you are moving to a city where there are multiple opportunities and you would not have to relocate if the first position turned out not to be permanent.

Of course, clinics and hospitals want you to buy a home so that they will have you more grounded and you will have a major reason not to move away. This is called "golden handcuffs," and it is in their best interest, because they do not want physician turnover. Many of them will actually help you arrange to buy a home with no down payment. This can be a great help to physicians. But for newly practicing physicians, it is not a reasonable option because you will pay huge amounts of interest for years to come. Further, you need to use your cash to pay off all your other debt quickly, not to buy a house with the first job and risk losing a great deal of money. As a newly practicing physician, you will probably earn a higher income than 95% of other Americans. At such a high income, you should then spend only 3 to 5 years to get totally out of debt, at the same time finding out if this first job is right for you long-term, and perhaps go on to become a young millionaire. Unfortunately, most physicians pay off their school loans over many years and continually borrow money for houses, cars, and credit cards. Over a 10-year period, paying a quarter of a million dollars or more in fees and interest to the lenders is not unusual. Hundreds of thousands of physicians stay in debt for most or all of their lives.

An interesting book on the subject is *The Millionaire Next Door* (Stanley and Danko 1996), also available on audiocassette. This best-selling book is based on careful research and outlines who the millionaires are in America. As the authors point out, physicians have been among the highest income earners in our nation since World War II, yet a disproportionately small number of them become independently wealthy, and most have to work long into their later years for financial reasons. Their biggest loss of wealth is due to acquiring large debts and then paying huge amounts in interest and fees, instead of keeping their own money to live a dramatically enhanced lifestyle while investing much of it for extreme wealth accumulation. To the contrary, far less educated people who earned much less than the average physician make up the overwhelming majority of our nation's self-made wealthy. Another best-selling book that outlines how to amass wealth (and why not to buy a house at first) is *Rich Dad, Poor Dad* (Kiyosaki 2000); it too is available on audiocassette. Perhaps the best motivator (to not spend all of one's money and still borrow more) is to remind the young physician of his or her children's future needs and to point out that the independently wealthy are able to provide for their children and live a life of much less stress and much more freedom than those who are not financially secure.

## Deciding What Is Important to You

As you are considering your career options and where you want to live, it is important to do your planning as discussed here. It is certainly not all about money. You are consciously choosing the lifestyle you desire, professionally and personally. This planning should be done with careful thought and introspection, and, if applicable, with involvement of your significant other. It does not have to be difficult. Appendix 2–A is a simple form that may be helpful.

This simplified approach to your initial planning should enable you to clarify which practice settings you plan to consider and to lay aside the many other opportunities that exist. This process also allows you to establish minimums, such as the minimum amount of money you must be able to make, the practicing setting you must have, and the part of the country in which you must live.

Notice that in section 2 of the form, you are asked to decide on a first, second, and third geographical choice. Perhaps the first choice is a particular city, the second is the state, and the third is contiguous states. Remember to strongly consider the place that you and your spouse call home.

In section 3, you can define not only the practice type, but also the income and benefits you desire (within reason). The practice opportunities offering an array of benefits will normally be those with large organizations, including hospitals and universities. Also be sure to write down the practice setting you do *not* want. Again, this helps you focus on the professional lifestyle you desire and prevent being burdened later by poor choices.

Section 4 asks how much money you really need in order to have a good lifestyle. If you earn $40,000 as a resident, perhaps after graduation you could have a fine lifestyle at $65,000 per year. In the United States, that is considered to be a very good income. You probably have a negative net worth now (that is, you owe more than you have in assets). By maintaining a moderate lifestyle like most Americans for just a few years, you then catapult yourself into the class that has no debt and a six-figure income. Your wealth can then go into buying a beautiful home (even if you then finance much of it), or buying your own office building, or investing in stocks and bonds, or establishing a 529 plan for your children's education, or taking time off, or donating to your favorite charities. Once you are debt free, your wealth grows rapidly and dramatically.

## Assessing the Opportunity

It is often a great surprise to young physicians to find they have chosen a position that does not work out, through no fault of their own. Many positions do not even last a full year. For this reason, it is of the utmost importance to check out the opportunity and the physicians.

Just as the practice or clinic will check your references, you should check theirs. Talking to their current physicians is a start, but the staff can be just as important. Get a feel for how well the practice or department is run. Is it well organized? Are certain managed care contracts or companies a problem? If physicians have resigned, find out why. The list of questions can be endless, but we advise you to trust your instincts. Think of each stage in terms of green, yellow, or red flags—go, caution, or stop. If the answers to your questions raise yellow flags, then ask more questions. If all is green, then proceed.

If you are seriously considering the position, your job is to ascertain whether the practice is as good as it seems and then to make a decision to keep pursuing it or to walk away. This fact-finding process can greatly affect your expectations so that you walk in with your eyes open and are not blindsided by new information that affects your job. For example, if the payer mix is largely managed care, are you being hired because of the additional managed care contract the practice has obtained? What happens if the contract is lost? Will you be the last in and first out?

You can also ask for the financial information on your new partners or employer—as your predecessors will have done in past years. The practice will have "financials," which include information such as the income statement, profit and loss statement, balance sheet, cash statement, and accounts aging report. Although a detailed discussion of this aspect is beyond the scope of this chapter, it is advisable to have someone knowledgeable look at such data to help you understand the numbers. If the practice hesitates, ask them what they would like to share, and mention that you understand providing financial information for new physicians considering a position is very common. You might need to tell them that it is all right to remove the actual salaries or other confidential information. If they will show you the financial information only in their office, ask if you can have their manager sit down with you to explain it. You can also have your own accountant or other professional go over the figures by phone to give you peace of mind or to identify problems you need to know about, such as hidden debt. Although more and more practices are readily providing such data, others are worried about this information being shared with the wrong person. Note, however, that the strongest, best-managed organizations take just the opposite stance. They are pleased to have someone interested and educated enough to ask such questions. Those who will not provide financial data of any sort definitely raise a red flag. Those who give limited information rate at least a yellow flag for the moment, but do not walk away too quickly.

With a private practice, when you are at the stage of asking for financial information you should always run a credit report on the business, just as many prospective employers are going to run a credit report on you. To check out the practice, go to the Internet address http://www.dnb.com. This is the Web site for Dun and Bradstreet, the nation's primary credit reporting company for businesses. At this writing, there are three levels of reports. We recommend the mid-level, which costs about $100. The basic level does not give enough information, and the advanced level is difficult to read. The mid-level report offers good information in the form of outlining whether or not the practice pays its bills on a timely basis. Don't worry if all the bills are not paid within 30 days. But if the practice routinely takes over 45 days to pay, that is a yellow flag. Over 60 days is a red flag. Remember, a yellow flag tells you to ask more questions, so don't become easily discouraged. There may be a good reason for the delay, such as difficulty in getting the managed care plans to pay faster—or you may have uncovered the tip of a financial nightmare. If you want to find a reputable professional consultant for assistance in evaluating Dun and Bradstreet credit reports and other aspects of a practice's performance, there are hundreds of consultants nationwide, and some can be extremely helpful at a reasonable cost. One might ask for referrals from other physicians. One might also look to consultants who are nationally known for writing books and articles and for teaching at conferences; these professionals are able to communicate clearly and tend to be the most interested in helping young physicians.

## Finding Opportunities

Again, your task is not only to find a position, but to find the position that is best for you personally and professionally, that pays what you want, and that is in the location you most desire. Most young doctors just fall into the "best" position that presents itself.

The key to finding good career opportunities is to be proactive and to start at least a year before graduation. The best positions are taken early on. So when you see something of interest, move quickly, because it probably will not be available for long.

Be careful not to listen to those who claim that the best positions are not advertised or promoted in any way and therefore are inaccessible. Many times those not advertised are indeed the best positions—and all you have to do is apply for the job.

To find your best career opportunities, we strongly recommend that you continue true networking—but not rely on it exclusively as many do. Networking is the process of asking who knows of a position, or where the need for a psychiatrist may be, and then calling or e-mailing the proper person directly. Mailing a letter when you hear of a position is usually not effective, except for academic positions that have a more formal hiring system. Sending an e-mail may net some result, but making a phone call is much better.

Go to the career center of the American Psychiatric Association (APA) for outstanding help in finding a position. You can post your curriculum vitae and also search job postings. Attend the annual meeting and visit the booths for those who are recruiting psychiatrists. Remember, there are plenty of opportunities. You just want the one that is best for you.

Next, comb the APA and other psychiatry publications for recruitment advertisements and follow up promptly. Ads also appear in non–specialty-specific publications, such as *JAMA*, *New England Journal of Medicine*, and *Medical Economics*. All of these journals also have the jobs posted on their Web sites, often before the magazine is published. If you get to those advertised positions first, you have a much better chance of being interviewed.

Opening your mail and quickly reviewing the recruitment pieces received can also present fine opportunities. If you have done the basic planning recommended here, this should be a quick and simple task. If the location is what you prefer, and if the practice setting is appropriate, respond immediately.

Accepting phone calls from recruiters may offer you the opportunity you desire. Remember there are search firm recruiters (headhunters) and employee in-house recruiters. The in-house recruiter is employed by the clinic, hospital, or health maintenance organization to find qualified, interested physicians. Many of these recruiters will call you after doing careful research. They may already have your curriculum vitae from the APA or another service, and they may be calling on behalf of a physician who has asked them to locate you. Search firms may be less desirable, but if you do take recruiters' calls, we advise you to quickly take control of the conversation and ask the questions that will tell you if there is an opportunity that fits your needs (such as the practice setting and the location of the practice or hospital). If the job does not meet your needs, you can be off the phone in 60 seconds. If it does meet your needs, then the possibility is open, even if you ask the recruiter to call you back or e-mail you. In any case, once you have established contact for a position of interest, get past the recruiter and speak with the physicians or administrators. The best recruiters want that, too.

Using Internet sites set up specifically to list physician opportunities

TABLE 2–1. Key words for Internet search

| Physician | + | Physician | + | City and/or state | + | Practice |
|---|---|---|---|---|---|---|
| Medical staff | | | | | | Opportunities |
| Doctor | | | | | | Placement |
| | | | | | | Search |
| | | | | | | Recruitment |
| | | | | | | Jobs |
| | | | | | | Positions |

can be an easy way to find positions. They charge a fee to the clinics and other employers who post the jobs, and there is no charge to you. There are many such sites, including these three that may be of interest:

- http://www.PracticeChoice.com
- http://www.PracticeLink.com
- http://web.medbulletin.com/Webodrome/jobHome.php

Searching the Internet can help you find more positions. Use the key words shown in Table 2–1. For best results, choose one word from each of the four columns. Currently, Google appears to be the best search engine for this purpose.

Going to physician recruitment exhibits can also present good opportunities. You may go to a national APA meeting or attend a state meeting. Also check what is available in your present area or in the area to which you want to move. Often there are recruitment fairs within a particular state that you may not hear about unless you search the Internet or make contact by e-mail or telephone. Possible contacts include the APA district branch, the state medical society, and city or county medical societies.

## ▌ DEALING WITH PROSPECTIVE EMPLOYERS

### How Much Are You Going to Pay Me?

Regarding how much a position pays: With search firms, we recommend that you ask that question right away. With all others, be very careful. If you have called to inquire about a position, or if the employers have called you or e-mailed you, it may not be in your best interest to ask about pay during the first conversation. After your curriculum vitae has been forwarded, and perhaps after they have sent you information, then if they do not bring up the subject of pay it's entirely appropriate to ask, if it is done properly. You definitely should ask before you travel across the country for an interview. If you are traveling only across town, or an hour away, perhaps you will wait until you meet them in person for the interview.

A proper way of putting the question might be, "By the way, can you give me an idea of the approximate range of pay a psychiatrist might earn in this position? Is there a production bonus on top of that? Can you tell me about the benefits?" Notice how the first question is asked with various qualifiers for a more gingerly approach to the question—words like "give me an idea," "approximate range," "might earn." The way you ask is paramount to obtaining the information without offending.

## Prepare for Your Site Visit and Interview

Some organizations will almost immediately ask you to come for an interview. Others may want to consider many candidates before they respond to you and may even conduct basic credentialing and background checks before meeting you in person.

From the hiring organization's perspective, there are two purposes for the visit. The first is to interview you to see if you may be the right person for them, and the second is to put their best foot forward to convince you to take the position. If you are interviewing locally or within a few hours' drive, these two functions may be broken out into separate visits. If you are interviewing from further away and staying overnight, the one visit probably includes both functions.

You will want to visit only those locations in which you have substantial interest, so choose carefully and prepare yourself as much as possible. You may start your preparation by asking various questions about the practice, department, hospital, fellow psychiatrists, and referring physicians. Ask the organization to send you as much information as possible about itself and the community. You should have one or more conversations with physicians by telephone. Do your research on the Internet as well. If you have to, take this information with you on the plane and read it there. Be sure to ask what to wear. Some will expect a nice dress or suit, so dress the part. You may need to purchase clothing and shoes for the occasion.

Be sure you have asked good questions prior to the interview, and be prepared to ask many more questions when you are there. This is no time to be quiet, even if that is your usual style. Also, realize that you need to put your best foot forward. At this point, humility is highly overrated. If you don't tell them you are a fine psychiatrist, your competition may very well get the job.

If your significant other will be going with you, coach him or her to ask good questions also, possibly about the community. If your significant other will be looking for a job in the vicinity, ask ahead of time if he or she can interview at a couple of places during the visit. Dual spouse recruitment is very common, and the employer may be happy to set up courtesy interviews in your spouse's field.

After the interview, follow up with at least an e-mail to say thank you. Or you may prefer to write a letter. Ideally, write each of the decision makers, or at least the key person such as the group's senior physician or the department head.

If you think you may want the position, be sure to ask at the end of the visit what the next step is. When you write or call afterwards, politely ask this question again to keep the ball rolling and to give you an idea what to expect.

## Avoid the Process of Elimination

Although the interview is one way for the organization to screen out candidates, there are other screens that you should be aware of, and some may be done even before you interview. Screens may include the following:

- *Credentialing.* This, of course, includes the verification of your education, licensure, and Drug Enforcement Administration number and a check of the National Practitioner Data Bank. Years ago this was thought to be all that was needed. But today there is much more.
- *Credit check.* A permission form will be presented to you to sign for this check. The employers want to find out whether you are a responsible person and whether there are any yellow or red flags because you evidently have personal financial problems. If you have any adverse history, be sure to tell them before they run the report; this will minimize the negative information. It is best to check your own credit ahead of time.
- *Criminal and civil courts checks.* These are two separate court systems in our country, and an organization will often have both checked for all the states and counties where you have lived to see if you have been convicted of crimes or involved in lawsuits.
- *Driver's license check.* The organization will be primarily looking for drug and alcohol abuse, but also for multiple speeding or other driving tickets. Again, they do not want to hire someone who is a "problem."
- *Professional and personal references.* You may be asked for three of each. Although you may coach your referees in what to say, if the employers think the references sound too coached or if they perceive any yellow flags, they will seek additional references as well.

- *Physical and drug screenings.* The larger organizations are routinely requiring these screenings. Smaller organizations usually do not.
- *Malpractice carriers check.* The organization will check your current and past carriers, with your permission, to see what litigation may have occurred.
- *Workers compensation check.* Here the employers will be looking at public and insurance company records, with your permission, to see if you have taken time off for workers comp.

### Get It in Writing

We have all heard that one must "get it in writing or it does not exist." For a newly hired physician, this applies as well. We strongly recommend asking that all salient points be addressed in writing, as part of the contract. If it feels uncomfortable to request this, then ask for confirmation in the form of a letter or e-mail. If this is still not appropriate, and if you are going to accept the position, then write an acceptance letter saying you are accepting the position based on this understanding. Ask them to respond to you by a certain day if this is not their understanding. And above all, be courteous, professional, and grateful for the opportunity they are affording you.

## ■ CONCLUSION

The opportunities for newly graduated psychiatrists abound. With private practice positions in every region of the country, it is not a matter of finding a position, but of finding the best position for each physician. In this chapter, I have reviewed the need for careful planning and for considering the various practice settings that are available, including going solo. The first position, on average, will last 2.4 years. Therefore it is imperative to make careful decisions regarding which position to take and not to overspend on housing and other significant expenditures.

The initial planning process can be simplified with the planning form provided in this chapter, and this process should identify the geographic areas and practice settings of interest. Finding the best position may be as simple as networking, but often it will be a result of searching the Internet, responding to advertisements and recruitment letters, and speaking with search firms and in-house recruiters.

A strong word of caution to the physician candidate is to consider carefully the pros and cons of each practice and community. Researching on the Internet and asking good questions can help in this regard. Obtaining a Dun and Bradstreet credit report on the private practice is recommended.

A professional who is experienced in such matters should review the contract and related financial information.

The best positions will probably have numerous applicants, so the interviewing physician should prepare carefully and realize that the clinic or hospital may conduct a background check that includes a credit check, a driver's license check, and more.

# ▌ REFERENCES

Bonds RG: National Physician Career Survey Report. Atlanta, GA, American Academy of Medical Management, 2004

Kiyosaki RT: Rich Dad, Poor Dad. New York, Warner Books, 2000

Stanley JT, Danko WD: The Millionaire Next Door. Atlanta, GA, Longstreet Press, 1996

## APPENDIX 2-A

# Planning Your Career Search

(If you have a significant other, all questions must be considered for both parties.)

1. Where are the jobs currently? Geographically and in practice setting type?

   _____

   _____

   _____

2. Identification of the geographic setting you prefer.

   First choice: _____

   Second choice: _____

   Third choice: _____

   List states or regions you do NOT want to live in:

   _____

   _____

3. What type of practice setting and income do you desire (i.e., six-physician free-standing group @$110,000 plus reasonable benefits and income potential, or full-time employment with large managed care company @$95,000 with full benefits and limited hours and call)?

   | Practice Setting | Income |
   |---|---|
   | First choice: _____ | $_____ |
   | Second choice:_____ | $_____ |
   | Third choice:_____ | $_____ |

   Type of practice setting you do NOT want:_____

4. What is the least amount of money you need to make to pay off bills and live the lifestyle you prefer? $_____

   (Don't forget cost of living differences in the offers you consider.)

# 3

# THE MANY FACES OF PRIVATE PRACTICE

*Jeremy A. Lazarus, M.D.*

After you have made the decision to enter private practice, it also makes good sense to consider the numerous types of private practice that are available. Although many people have an image of the individual psychiatrist in a single office with a waiting room, that is not the only type of private practice available. Indeed, there are many forms of private practice that open up a range of opportunities for those starting on this course. In this chapter, I'll discuss the advantages and disadvantages of some different practice arrangements, the likely types of patients in various settings, subspecialty influence, physician networks, and lifestyle issues.

## ■ PRACTICE SETTINGS

There are five general practice settings in the private sector:

1. Solo practice
2. Small psychiatric group
3. Large psychiatric group
4. Multidisciplinary group
5. Multispecialty group

## Solo Practice

First, and still the most common for private practice psychiatry, is the solo office-based psychiatric practice. Solo practice has a number of distinct advantages. One is the complete autonomy that you have in solo practice. You call all the shots regarding where and when to practice, how much to work, how to arrange your office, and any other details about your professional life. When changes need to be made in any of these, it's you who ultimately decides. So decisions and changes that are made are always consistent with what you value. A corollary advantage is that you have control over which patients, and how many patients, to serve. Some psychiatrists will choose to see only individual patients in psychotherapy, or in psychotherapy and medication management, whereas some will choose to have a psychopharmacology practice only, leaving psychotherapy to others. Some psychiatrists will see a mix of individual patients, couples, families, and groups. You can make these choices on the basis of needs in the community served and also according to your competencies.

Another advantage of solo practice is that you have both business and financial control over your practice. All of your decisions are your own, made by yourself or with advice from family, friends, or consultants. You decide how to set up the business, billing, and accounting aspects of your practice. You also have authority over all of these functions, and it is your responsibility to know what is happening on the business side of your practice. This business oversight will affect your income and expenses, and you will be in the best position to know the details of what is going on financially.

You will also determine whether or not to hire any office staff. In a busy practice, it is often quite helpful to have part-time or full-time staff to perform general office duties such as answering the phone, opening mail, and keeping up with other regular office details. Of course, staff assistance comes with a cost, but in the long run it may save you time to be more productive in your income-generating work.

The final advantage of solo practice is the ease of change. If you believe change is warranted, it's your decision whether to move offices, change staff, alter the patient mix, or change any number of other parameters of practice.

On the other hand, there are also some disadvantages to solo practice. Mentioned by many is the relative isolation that comes with private practice. After one has finished residency training or work in another type of setting, a solo private practice can be very isolating. Although there can be great pleasure and satisfaction in treating patients hour after hour, many people also like the ability to interact with colleagues for professional or social reasons. The more physically isolated the solo office, the more potential there is for isolation from other people. Breaking up the practice day with activities that involve others can mitigate this, but it does take planning and is not part of the everyday office experience. Some enjoy the full patient day and reserve their professional interactions for evening meetings. In short, there are ways to augment professional interaction, but it takes some effort.

One final disadvantage is the relatively increased fixed costs of a solo practice. Because all expenses are borne by one person, your staff, billing, phone, accounting, faxing, rent, and all other office-based expenses are your responsibility. Although you may have better control as an individual, you may find that these practice expenses eat away too much of your income.

## Small Psychiatric Group

A small psychiatric group, for purposes of this discussion, is from two to four psychiatrists. There are a number of advantages to this type of practice arrangement. First, there is the opportunity for collaboration, either in a formal way or in the time-honored "curbside consultation." When two to four psychiatrists share an office suite, they will inevitably come across each other in the waiting room, in the hallway, or in their administrative space. Although discussions about patient issues need to be carefully monitored so that there are no confidentiality breaches, it's very easy in the small group practice to go next door and ask a question, get a scientific update, or keep up your personal relationship. Some small group practices set up regular scientific practice updates by either having a journal club, inviting in guest speakers, or doing their own case presentations.

Another advantage to a small psychiatric group is the ability to share fixed costs like office rent, waiting room space, office staff, and office equipment and telephone or other business services. Some small psychiatric groups have also invested in their own buildings, which they use for their own practices or rent out to other professionals. A small psychiatric group also may be better able to negotiate with third-party payers for fees or payment terms than an individual psychiatrist might.

If there are good working and professional relationships in the small group, the possibilities for interoffice referral are very high. When one member of the group is too busy or thinks another can handle a particular case better, it is far easier to chat with someone down the hall than to call someone outside the office to make the referral. Knowing and respecting each other's abilities will of course determine the extent of interoffice referral, but this possibility does not exist in the solo practice. It also may be easier to set up cross-coverage with others within this office setting than it might be if you needed to find colleagues outside the office.

There are also some disadvantages to small group practice. Because decision making is shared, time must be set aside to reach consensus on important business or practice choices. The ability to compromise is definitely a desirable attribute, and without it, this type of arrangement is doomed. If you're fiercely independent and it's no way but your way, then don't go this route.

You also need to keep in mind that there may be increased investment costs in a small group practice. The group may decide to purchase office equipment that is either more complicated or more expensive than the type you would purchase as an individual. You may need to consider investing in a building, providing benefits for office staff, or making other financial commitments that would not exist in a solo practice. Once you're in this type of practice, extracting yourself may be cumbersome, and you may be obligated to financial expenditures that you hadn't expected.

## Large Psychiatric Group

Here I am referring to any group above four. The advantages are an extension of those in small group practice. The ability to have greatly increased collaboration among colleagues is an advantage. Many larger psychiatric groups will have members with varying expertise in subspecialty practice, with the result that intraoffice referral is greatly heightened. Of course, with the increased numbers come increased opportunities for on-the-spot consultation on patient care questions.

With increased numbers comes the ability to share fixed office costs with a larger group and ideally be more cost-efficient for each member. Spreading the financial risks among more individuals should ultimately lessen individual expenses. The larger the group, the greater the ability to negotiate with payers. In addition, office staff will be a necessity, and costs can be shared.

With the larger group, however, comes the increased time it takes to maintain the collaboration, especially for the business side of the practice. Issues related to how decisions are made in a large group and the complexities of group dynamics begin to play a role. Think of group conflicts in your residency or medical school and you can be sure that some types of group conflicts will play themselves out in this setting as well. To get you through the tough times, it's important to have good processes in place, good professional relationships, a good sense of humor, and at least some social appreciation of each other. Good and binding ties are necessary when thorny issues come up. For example, if you all own a building together, make sure that your partnership agreement will stand any kind of test in the event of a partner's death, disability, retirement, or wish to sell. Having a trusted attorney picked by the group for these purposes is critical.

With the larger group comes the potential for larger investment costs.

If you're part of the large group and they decide to purchase a computer system that you think is too costly, you may need to go along with the decision even though you don't totally agree. Compromise, negotiation, and good interpersonal processes get large groups through these thorny dilemmas.

With a larger group, the ease of change also diminishes. Because you need to assess the wishes and needs of a larger group, changes may come more slowly than you might like. This can either work for or against you in the end.

## Multidisciplinary Group Practice

Here I am referring to a mental health professional group consisting of a mix of psychiatrists, psychologists, social workers, and nursing practitioners or others. In such a group, there will be multiple opportunities for interoffice referral and collaboration. Often in such a group, the psychiatrists may take on the more complex psychopharmacology cases and collaborate with the other professionals who are doing psychotherapy while the psychiatrist is providing the medication management services.

There is no one ideal model in such an arrangement, and some of these practices just grow over time as professionals get to know each other in the community or when they work closely together on cases. The range of services that can be provided in such a group practice is significantly greater than in a psychiatry-only practice. Often, therapeutic modalities may be provided by the other professionals that are not part of the usual psychiatrist's armamentarium. The opportunity to do conjoint treatment or co-lead groups is another possibility.

The advantage of sharing of fixed costs is present, but this may become more complicated with a different mix of professionals. For example, the psychiatrists might want to have a nurse available to draw blood for laboratory tests, whereas the non-M.D. professionals might not find this a good investment. The other potential business advantage of this type of group is the ability to provide a place for "one-stop shopping" for all mental health services (assuming you offer most of them). Your group may be able to represent itself to third-party payers, referring physicians, and others as a place where almost any type of patient can be referred and treated.

With the increased size, however, come some potential disadvantages. There will inevitably be increased time for collaboration and decision making. If you are in an employer or supervisory relationship with some of the other professionals, there are increased legal, ethical, and business ramifications. Consultation with a good practice attorney, accountant, and/or business consultant will be critical. If you all share in decision making, then there may be group dynamic issues. Again, the need for compromise and consensus is essential to success.

In addition, the complexity from a business point of view necessitates that at least several members of the group have some business or financial skills to make sure that your business decisions are sound. It may make sense, if the group is large enough, to hire an office manager with these skills to manage the routine business issues while the professionals provide guidance and oversight. All of these points of decision may involve costs or investment, and you should be prepared to approach a multidisciplinary group with the appropriate questions to see whether it fits in with your style and interests.

## Multispecialty Group

I am referring here to a group made up of mental health professionals as well as physicians or professionals from other specialties. In addition to all of the advantages of the multidisciplinary group, this type of practice offers possibilities for more integrated care of patients. This might be advantageous especially for patients with comorbid medical problems, those with chronic illnesses, or complicated cases requiring multiple specialists. Such a practice will inevitably have a more "medical" feel to it, but for a psychiatrist who enjoys working with complicated cases and working closely with other physicians, this may be an ideal practice situation. In addition, the opportunities for ongoing collaboration and medical education will undoubtedly be increased. Such a setting exponentially increases the opportunities for "curbside consult," referrals, and practice-building.

If you enter such a practice as a co-owner or partner, you will have the benefits of sharing broader and perhaps more efficient practice expenses. A multispecialty group will also have increased clout in contracting with payers and may be able to present opportunities for education, research, and practice incentives that may not be available in a smaller practice. A multispecialty group will usually have good business support services that relieve the professionals in the group from the business burdens of a smaller practice.

With the larger size, however, may come some disadvantages. It may be difficult in such a setting to say no to a referral, so your ability to control your patient type and flow may be diminished. In addition, you will have much less financial control as a member of a large group, and your voice will be only one of many. Other specialists may have other needs resulting in costs to the group that you would not ordinarily invest in if your practice were strictly psychiatric. For example, there may be imaging services that may generate a cost to you but for which you have limited needs. Your professional and business autonomy will then be captive to a much larger degree to the larger group, and you will have to be prepared to adjust.

The business and financial decision making of this type of group will also be more complex, and the time to oversee, review, and come to consensus may be substantially greater than in the other types of practices.

As you think about the types of private practice and whether any of these are particularly appealing to you, make sure that you find psychiatrists in these types of practices to talk to. Ask them tough questions about their views of the advantages and disadvantages, what they would have done differently, what you should look out for, and whether they would do it this way again.

## ■ PATIENT/PRACTICE TYPE

It's important to recognize that there is no "one size fits all" in private practice. One can do outpatient, inpatient, consultation, evaluation, and any other number of combinations of these types of work in practice.

Although this book will not attempt to cover the range of subspecialties, it is also important to recognize that different subspecialties in psychiatry may put their own stamp on a private practice. For example, if you're a child psychiatrist, you'll likely need a different office setup with a playroom. If you are a geriatric psychiatrist, you may want to have special provisions in your waiting room, or you may need office staff to assist the elderly with filling out forms or interacting with other treating physicians. If you're a forensic psychiatrist, it's possible that much of your work will be done away from your office, for example in a jail or prison. If you're a consulting psychiatrist, much of your work may be done in the hospital. All of these examples illustrate the complex and multifaceted nature of private practice and the need for careful research and advice on determining the best practice milieu and setup for you.

## ■ PHYSICIAN NETWORKS

There are many varieties of networks that psychiatrists can join either for referral purposes or as a provider. The types of physician networks are independent practice associations (IPAs), preferred provider organizations (PPOs), health maintenance organizations (HMOs), and behavioral health companies or carveouts. All of these entities have advantages and disadvantages for psychiatrists.

In brief, the more integrated the network (such as integrated patient records, outcomes, or coordinated care), the more you will have the advantages and disadvantages of integration. The more integrated the network, the less autonomous you are, but you also may benefit from economies of scale, negotiating clout, and contract management that will not be available if you're in a smaller practice. Much information is available to psychiatrists on the American Psychiatric Association Web site at http://www.psych.org/psych_pract/. The American Medical Association has considerable information through its Web site at http://www.ama-assn.org. On that site, look under "Professional Resources" for "Practice mgmt. tools." An excellent model managed care contract is also available at that site under "Professional Resources." State medical societies usually have information available to help practicing clinicians with information pertinent to that state (and may also require membership). A thorough understanding of the benefits and risks of joining one of these organizations is critical. We have seen over and over that psychiatrists and other physicians will sign contracts without reading them thoroughly or getting legal advice, will accept fee structures that they are uncertain about, and will not take advantage of any negotiating ability they may have. Remember, talk to more experienced colleagues, research the network, and don't sign contracts for networks without understanding the nature of your resultant obligations.

# ▎ LIFESTYLE ISSUES

As you think about the type of practice setting that you want to work in, you should also make a careful assessment of how your practice choice will influence your personal life. The practice settings described in this chapter also have effects on one's personal life, ranging from the ultimate flexibility of the solo practice to the potential complexities of a multispecialty group's demands. Remember that your autonomy diminishes as you increase the numbers of people you work with. Although you many enjoy the cross-coverage in a larger group, you may also dislike the increase in the number of calls you have to take when you're on call. If you are doing a more predominantly hospital consulting or medical clinic type of practice, you may need to be more immediately available to go to the hospital or clinic and possibly interrupt your day. Likewise, if you have a mix of outpatients and inpatients, you may need to juggle your schedule regularly to make things work.

As mentioned in the introductory chapter, there are multiple opportunities to interact with other psychiatrists and physicians when you enter practice. You are usually invited to attend grand rounds or other educational opportunities at your local university medical center. You can take advantage of hospital, medical society, or psychiatric society educational meetings. If you are interested in volunteering, there are numerous places where your services would be welcomed, such as in clinics for the homeless, clinics or services for the uninsured, and services through religious organizations. You will always be welcomed to join activities through county or state medical societies or the district branch of the APA.

If you have a particular interest in the political aspects of health care, there are the possibilities for physicians to take training through the American Medical Association Political Action Committee (AMPAC) on how to run a political campaign. You can learn more about these programs at their Web site: http://www.ampaconline.org. You can enrich your education and experience through various online educational programs leading to degrees in business, management, or finance. If, as part of a practice, you decide that you need more business education, you can seek further education through medical organizations or through college programs in your city.

Although time management can be tricky, don't stop learning to improve your professional and business competencies. The key is to pick those educational activities that will make a real difference in your professional or business life. You should strive toward always being the best psychiatrist possible while improving your ability to make an adequate living with the least hassles.

To round out your volunteer activities, consider joining a committee, whether of a hospital staff you are on, through your county or state medical society, for your district branch of the American Psychiatric Association, or for your subspecialty organization. These organizations always need volunteers and involvement, and it will help you to keep in touch with psychiatrist and physician colleagues and benefit your profession. You might also consider leadership opportunities in these organizations if that's your bent. Finding professional activities to supplement your patient practice can make your professional life more fulfilling.

# █ CONCLUSION

I hope you can sense the broad range of possibilities that await you in private practice. The combinations that will lead to a gratifying professional life are endless, and you'll certainly need some time to find the combination that is right for you. It's also quite possible that you'll make a few changes in your practice setting as you sort through what works best for you.

Remember in the end that if you love what you do, you'll make the most of your training as a psychiatrist.

# 4 THE PSYCHIATRIC OFFICE

*Jonathan M. Kersun, M.D.*

*Edward K. Silberman, M.D.*

Setting up an office is an important and central aspect of getting started in private practice. This step in career development can seem forbidding and is often laden with anxiety. How is an office created when none currently exists? On the one hand, this is a very simple matter; one needs a small office with a waiting room, a phone, an appointment book, and malpractice insurance. Indeed, when conceptualized in this way, there is an elegant simplicity to the whole endeavor. On the other hand, there are a lot of practical details that need to be addressed as one plans and executes setting up an office. Moreover, setting up an office is usually a quantum jump toward autonomy. It can be frightening to separate from the familiar institutional setting of medical school and residency and create your own space. At the same time, having your own office can be an enormous source of pride and gratification. In this chapter we address the specifics of setting up an office in an effort to help the graduating resident pursue this process in a thoughtful and thorough fashion.

## ■ LOCATION

The area where you decide to practice is an important consideration; it is likely you will remain in that area for many years. It is important to be able to feel that this area is a place where you would enjoy working. Here a little bit of research and some careful thought go a long way. Choosing an area in which to practice is not unlike choosing a significant other; there is a chemistry and compatibility that, when present, go a long way toward helping a practice flourish. You need to consider, also, whether the area is a place where you would enjoy living. Enjoying the location will positively affect the growth and development of the practice.

Many complex factors are involved in choosing where to practice. Some were noted in earlier chapters: Do you have a commitment to a particular area? Do you like a rural, a suburban, or an urban setting? Is a particular geography and climate preferable? There are other factors as well: Is the population of a particular area going to be able to support the type of practice you want to establish? A fee-for-service psychotherapy practice usually requires a different socioeconomic milieu than an insurance-based practice. Ongoing fee-for-service psychotherapy is expensive; a patient needs to be psychologically amenable to and financially able to pay for his or her treatment. Many patients are not so inclined, even if the therapist is willing to be flexible with the fee. Therefore, a fee-for-service psychotherapy practice, in all likelihood, needs an upper middle class population base in order to develop successfully. Similar considerations apply if you are setting up a general psychiatric practice. Because patients in a general psychiatric practice tend to be seen less frequently, the cost burden to the patient tends to be less. Therefore, it is probably somewhat easier to establish a fee-for-service general psychiatric practice. However, if you are planning on accepting insurance, the socioeconomic milieu of your office is less of a pressing concern.

There are other questions that need to be asked as well. What is the psychiatric community in the area like—is it collegial and collaborative, or is it more competitive and turf oriented? In general, it is a good idea to call several psychiatrists in the area that you are considering and speak with them about their practices. Learn about how they practice: How frequently are patients seen? What is the length of a session? How much of what is done is pharmacologically oriented versus psychotherapeutically oriented? If psychotherapy is practiced, what type or types? Do the physicians have good relationships with the other psychiatrists in the area? Ask them whether they take insurance and if so, which plans. Inquiring about fee structures can be a delicate subject. Some colleagues will volunteer this information in an effort to be helpful to you; others will not. You can safely ask good friends and recent graduates about what they charge to get a sense of pricing. Ask other psychiatrists if they have employees and what the employees do for them. How much do they pay for rent? If someone is resistant to answering these questions, the individual might feel threatened by new competition. Encountering resistance from several psychiatrists will tell you a lot about the psychiatric milieu in the area.

You need to know what kinds of resources are available for psychiatric hospitalization and where patients are referred for crisis intervention. It is a good idea to consider what kinds of public transportation are available in a given area. In an urban setting, it is quite possible patients will need or want to use public transportation to get to your office. You might consider an office location near a train or subway stop. Even in suburban practices, patients might wish to get to your office by train or bus if this is an option. Another good thing is to check out the medical hospitals in an area. See how many psychiatrists are on staff. If many psychiatrists are already practicing in an area, that is not a contraindication to opening an office; it is merely a variable to consider. The truth of the matter is that a good and savvy psychiatrist will succeed no matter the degree of saturation; it might, however, take somewhat longer to become established. If you are relatively open-minded, ambitious, able to take advantage of opportunities when they are presented, dedicated to providing excellent care, patient, creative, and relatively flexible, you will likely succeed wherever you open your practice. Indeed, there is certain wisdom to the expression "If you build it, they will come."

## ❚ OFFICE

Once you have decided on a particular area, you then need to obtain a space in which to practice. You need your *own* office, quite an exciting idea. The options here are many. If you are considering joining the staff of a local hospital, there is often an office building associated with the hospital. Sometimes an office in such a building can be rented on a part-time basis. Also, there are usually physicians—not only psychiatrists—looking to sublet some of their space. One can rent one's own office in a medical office building, but this does tend to be quite expensive. You can get the information you need about such spaces by contacting the administration at the particular hospital. Having an office in such a building has the advantage of placing you directly in a medical community where you can easily get to know other physicians to begin to establish a base of referral. If you are going to be doing hospital consultation work, an office in a medical office building is extremely convenient; you can easily do a consultation in between patients. This milieu is also helpful from a social standpoint in that solo psychiatric practice can be somewhat isolating and lonely.

Another option for an office is a professional building. Most areas have many such buildings. This type of office can have the social and collegial advantage of the hospital medical office building, and it tends to be less expensive. One way to find out where these buildings are is to call the office of the local government—town hall or borough hall—and ask for a list. You can also simply drive or walk around a neighborhood that you like and that seems to be commercially oriented. Look for "office for lease" signs. Write down the number and give the person a call. It can be quite fun and surprising to explore and see what you learn.

If you want a less traditionally medical type of office, one that is more personal and homey, this random wandering around approach can often be quite fruitful. One of the authors came across many interesting options in this way. One such option was subleasing some space from a law office in a building from the Revolutionary War period. You might also consider renting a one-bedroom apartment and converting it into a psychiatric office. This option can be very affordable and provide space that is very attractive. It is always nice to have a kitchen in which to store lunch food, soda, and coffee. The advantages of this type of space are many. The space is distinctly private and does not have the "medical office" look. Patients often find this very comforting and appealing, which can be a good thing when you are trying to establish a place where people can feel at ease and trusting. This type of office also affords a lot of latitude in terms of how the space is decorated. It is important to ascertain, however, if zoning regulations in the particular location can permit medical practice. Again, the local government office can provide this information.

Another option is building or purchasing an office building or space. This can be done alone or with others. There are many advantages to owning your own space from a tax and investment standpoint. However, it is probably better to get settled into your new practice before entertaining the purchase of real estate. There is much to be learned in the initial years of practice; owning business real estate adds more to the already large pile of things that you need to learn and know about. After you have been in practice for several years, you might consider purchasing your own space. By this time you will be familiar with the area and will know other professionals with whom you might want to partner in a business venture.

Finally, if you purchase a home, having a home office is also a possibility, assuming that a portion of the home could be configured for such a purpose. In all likelihood a separate entrance will be required for patients, and there will need to be space that is dedicated specifically to the office so that the office boundaries are clear to both the patient and the psychiatrist. It can be extremely convenient to practice out of one's home, and it can be beneficial for patients to see that their doctor is a "real person." There are also significant tax advantages to having a home office; a portion of your mortgage, your phone line, snow removal, and even toilet paper and so forth, can be claimed as business expenses. Speak to an accountant and/or to a psychiatrist with a home office to learn about the specific tax regulations regarding a home office. There are also disadvantages to having a home office, particularly when you are first starting out. In the early stages of practice, many different types of patients will likely be coming through. You may not feel comfortable having patients with psychosis or severe personality disorders coming to a home office. Having a home office also requires psychological flexibility and comfort with being exposed. Establishing a practice after residency is a difficult endeavor; having a home office might be an added stress in an already stressful time. It is often better to get established for a while before undertaking a home office.

Sharing space with another psychiatrist is also a possibility. In getting to know the psychiatric community, you will often find that other psychiatrists have office space they would like to share or sublease. You can also share space with psychologists. Sharing space is usually less expensive than solo occupancy, but you have to deal the variables involved in having a "roommate." It can be nice to have someone to talk to and discuss cases with, but it can also be difficult if you do not get along with the other person or persons. Sharing space can be in the form of having your own office in a suite of offices or actually sharing an office, one person using the office when the other is not there. Although some don't mind sharing an office, it is generally more satisfying and comfortable to have space that you can call your own. It will help you feel settled and enhance your sense of receptivity, which is important when listening to patients.

The above options for office space and their advantages and disadvantages are summarized in Table 4–1.

After you have found space, you need to formalize the acquisition through execution of a lease. Most commercial space is leased for periods of time somewhat longer than the usual 1-year lease of residential spaces. It is often helpful to have an attorney review the lease agreement before signing. Often, attorneys can discern ways in which the lease might be worded to be more favorable to the tenant. Common difficulties arise in delineating responsibility for the physical space. Who is responsible for what in the event something breaks or malfunctions? What is reasonable wear and tear, as opposed to damage, to carpet, walls, and such? It should be clearly established who is responsible for payment of utilities. If the landlord is paying utilities, is there an escalation clause that the landlord can add on to your bill? It should be specified that the landlord is not permitted to enter the office without your permission and notification, unless there is an emergency such as fire or flood. You should establish a time frame within which the landlord is responsible to respond to requests from you. For example, if the toilet is broken, the landlord should be responsible for having it fixed within a reasonable period of time, say 24 to 48 hours.

TABLE 4–1.  Office space options

| Space option | Advantages | Disadvantages |
|---|---|---|
| Medical office building (attached to hospital) | • Proximity to medical community<br>• Convenient for C/L work<br>• Less lonely<br>• Can share space | • Expensive<br>• Potentially sterile appearance |
| Medical office building (unattached to hospital) | • Proximity to medical community<br>• Less lonely<br>• Can share space | • Expensive<br>• Potentially sterile appearance |
| Professional building | • Can meet other professionals<br>• Less expensive than medical office building | • Still relatively expensive<br>• Potentially sterile appearance |
| Residential/nonmedical building | • "Homey" atmosphere<br>• Affordable<br>• Usually quite private | • Lack of contact with potential referral sources<br>• Isolating |
| Construction of office | • Can customize to own needs<br>• Good investment<br>• Tax savings | • Expensive, particularly early on in career<br>• Many unknown variables to consider without adequate experience<br>• Potentially isolating |
| Home office | • Convenient<br>• Tax savings<br>• Personal atmosphere<br>• Usually quite private | • Diminished separation of personal and professional<br>• Concern with difficult patients in one's home<br>• Isolating |

*Note.*  C/L=consultation/liaison.

If for some reason damage occurs to the office at your hands, you should have the right to be involved in selecting who does the repairs. Otherwise, the landlord can bring in whomever he or she wants to repair the problem and charge you for it. You might consider adding a clause listing conditions under which you would be allowed to break the lease (i.e., if the landlord is not fulfilling stipulated obligations). Almost more important than the lease itself, however, is the relationship one has with one's landlord. If you get a good impression of the person (and if others say favorable things about him or her) and if you are able to forge a pleasant, amicable professional relationship, difficulties can be held to a minimum.

Often a lease will stipulate that the lessee (or tenant) must have liability insurance to cover both the tenant and the landlord in the event of an accident's happening to someone on the premises. This policy is fairly standard. The amount of coverage varies according to geographic area, and the insurance policy itself is fairly inexpensive.

# ▮ MONEY

You will need a certain amount of capital to set up a practice. Your yearly costs can vary tremendously, depending most significantly on your rent and malpractice costs. Many of your start-up costs will be one-time expenses; these too can vary enormously. An estimate of first-year expenses ranges from $18,650 to $75,550 in 2004 dollars (Table 4–2). Often, however, when finishing residency, you do not have much money; you may even be in significant debt. A number of options are available here. You can go to a local bank and apply for a line of credit. This is, for all intents and purposes, a loan, usually with quite a low interest rate. The bank will proffer an amount of money that will be available for your use. This money can be paid back over a period of time that is determined by the bank.

Another option is to place purchases for the practice on a credit card. Using credit cards can be done in a rather imaginative way. Most are familiar with the ubiquitous offers received in the mail for credit cards. Many of these offers are for very low rates; some actually have a 0% rate that will remain in place for 1 to 2 years. This amounts to an interest-free loan. If after the "loan period" is up one has not completed paying off the debt, one can then transfer the balance to another 0% card. You do, however, need to be diligent about paying down the balance and making sure you understand the specifics of the credit card so as to avoid "hidden" charges. Initial costs will include furniture, supplies, equipment, malpractice insurance, and a deposit for office space—usually first and last months' rent. If you are going to have staff, that will be another expense.

You need to establish a business checking account. You also need to create a bookkeeping system to track business expenses for accounting purposes. There are many inexpensive and relatively simple software programs, such as Quickbooks or Quicken, that can help in this regard.

TABLE 4–2. Start-up costs (for first year in practice)

| Item | Cost range ($) |
|------|----------------|
| Furniture | 2,500–5,000 |
| Decoration | 500–1,500 |
| Plants | 75–200 |
| Magazine subscriptions | 250–400/year |
| Computer equipment | 1,000–4,000 |
| Copy equipment | 200–400 |
| Phone equipment | 100–300 |
| Fax machine | 50–200 |
| Stationery, supplies, and medical record forms | 300–1,200 |
| Deposit for office space | 800–3,000 |
| Rent | 400–1,500/month |
| Cleaning service | 50–200/month |
| Billing service | 100–1,500/month |
| Hospital privileges | 200–800/year |
| Beeper | 75–150/year |
| Malpractice insurance | 6,000–20,000/year |
| *Range of total first-year expenditures* | 18,650–75,550 |

Some combine bookkeeping and check-writing functions. Another option is a One-write system, which is available from several office product companies (McBee, 800-662-2331; Histaccount, 800-645-5220). This system combines a checking register with a ledger page for bookkeeping. When you write a check, a carbon copy is recorded on the ledger page. You then record the check amount in a corresponding column. This system allows for easy tracking of all business-related expenses. Income from the practice can also be easily tracked as one's deposits to the account are recorded. Keeping a ledger card (a record of debits, credits, and balance) for each patient is also necessary.

If you are uncertain and have questions about this area of the practice, you can ask other psychiatrists what they do, or you can consult with an accountant who might be able to help establish the bookkeeping aspect of the practice from the outset. Bear in mind that all expenses related to the practice are tax deductible, including lunches that you have with colleagues to discuss your practice. Get in the habit of thinking about expenses as either practice-related or personal. An accountant can help you understand and take full advantage of what you are entitled to declare as practice-related expenses.

It is also a good idea to open a credit card account solely for the practice. Many credit card companies will send an expense breakdown at year's end. These breakdowns can be added to the running totals on one's master ledger sheet to itemize expenses for accounting. Get a credit card for which each dollar spent earns airline frequent flyer miles or some other type of bonus, and put as much of your practice expenses on the credit card as possible. Again, make sure to pay off the balance at month's end to avoid running into debt.

# ▌ BILLING

Generating income through practice is very unfamiliar territory for the newly graduated resident. Making your own way financially is both an exciting and a somewhat intimidating venture. You need to decide to what extent, if at all, you want to participate in insurance plans. Participation in various plans can allow a practice to grow faster, because many, many patients will use only their insurance as a means of payment for medical treatment. Speak to area psychiatrists and find out which insurance plans are most advantageous and physician friendly. Many health insurance providers subcontract their psychiatric benefits to behavioral health care companies. Some of these companies are easier to work with than others. Find out which behavioral companies provide services in your area and which of these are the most reasonable to work with. Medicare participation is often a safe bet because Medicare is not yet a managed care system. Reimbursement is reasonable, payment is prompt, and one does not have to deal with a lot of paperwork and limitations regarding patients. Call 866-488-0548 to obtain information about becoming a Medicare provider.

If you do not want to have insurance involvement, you can develop a fee-for-service practice. *This can be done.* A fee-for-service practice takes time to develop. It is part of the craft of psychiatry to learn, slowly, how to work with patients on the issue of payment. It helps here to be flexible. You can discuss with patients that the fee is a part of the treatment, that an amount needs to be charged that is reasonable for the patient—not so low as to be insulting, not so high as to be unaffordable, and reasonable to the doctor as well. Learning how to work in this manner can be quite rewarding and interesting.

A bill can be generated for the patient at the end of each month, or payment can be collected session by session. It can be helpful to have printed a form called a *superbill* (Figure 4–1). A superbill can be given to patients as a form of receipt that they can submit to their insurance companies, and it can also be used for billing if one is doing other types of practice such as hospital consultation or nursing home work.

## ∎ STAFF

You may or may not have a need to hire office staff. For psychiatry, office personnel can help with secretarial tasks, billing, and office management. Because of the expense involved in paying another's salary, many psychiatrists opt to hire office personnel only after they having been practicing for a while. If you envision a practice where patients are seen monthly or less often and where the focus is pharmacologic, it is likely that patient volume will be high. Here it might be helpful to have a person assist with scheduling, phoning in prescriptions, preparing bills, doing bookkeeping, typing letters, and helping with insurance company issues. Ask other psychiatrists and physician colleagues about how they hired their office staff and whether they know any good people. Inquire about the typical salary range for your particular geographic area. Speak to an accountant about the logistics of having an employee.

Often when psychiatrists are just starting out, going it alone can be efficient and cost-effective. In any case, it is generally a good idea to learn how to do your own office management so that when the time comes to hire someone, you know how your system works and you can teach it to your staff. If you are going to try to develop a more psychotherapeutically oriented practice where patients are seen more often and total patient volume is relatively low, you might be able to establish a practice without ever needing to hire anyone. It is usually possible to hire someone part-time on a fee-for-service basis to help with transcription and with bookkeeping. Usually, people who can provide this type of help do not need to work out of your office. Rather, they work from their own homes or places of business. Again, speak to your physician colleagues; they might be able to suggest people who are good and reasonably priced.

Hiring a billing company can be helpful, particularly if you are doing large-volume psychopharmacology, consultation/liaison, or nursing home work. A billing company works on the doctor's behalf to bill insurance companies or patients. It keeps track of outstanding balances and works to ensure that payments are made. Usually billing companies charge a percentage of payments received for their services, typically 6%–10%. Again, check with area doctors about local billing companies. Some companies specialize in psychiatric billing, and some do only nonpsychiatric billing.

JONATHAN M. KERSUN, M.D.
PSYCHIATRY

SUITE 2
110 PARK AVENUE
SWARTHMORE, PA 19081    (610) 543-2300

Date:_____

Patient Name:_____

| CPT | CODES | DESCRIPTION | CHARGE | | CPT | CODES | DESCRIPTION | CHARGE |
|---|---|---|---|---|---|---|---|---|
| x | | Psychotherapy Codes with Medication Mgmt | | | x | | Inpatient Consults | |
| | 90801 | Initial Psychiatric Evaluation | | | | 99251 | Initial Level I | |
| | 90862 | 15 Min Med Check | | | | 99252 | Initial Level II | |
| | 90805 | 20-30 Min E & M | | | | 99253 | Initial Level III | |
| | 90807 | 45-50 Min E & M | | | | 99254 | Initial Level IV | |
| | 90809 | 75-80 Min E & M | | | | 99255 | Initial Complex Comprehensive | |
| | | Psychotherapy Codes (Non Medication Mgmt) | | | | | Follow-up Inpatient Consults | |
| | 90804 | 20-30 Min Indiv Psychotherapy | | | | 99261 | Follow-up Level I | |
| | 90806 | 45-50 Min Indiv Psychotherapy | | | | 99262 | Follow-up Level II | |
| | 90808 | 75-80 Min Indiv Psychotherapy | | | | 99263 | Follow-up Level III | |
| | 90845 | Psychoanalysis | | | | 99231 | Hosp Subsequent I | |
| | | Office Consultations | | | | 99232 | Hosp Subsequent II | |
| | 99241 | Level I Office Consultation | | | | 99233 | Hosp Subsequent III | |
| | 99242 | Level II Office Consultation | | | | | Skilled Nursing Consults | |
| | 99243 | Level III Office Consultation | | | | 99301 | SNF Initial Eval Level I | |
| | 99244 | Level IV Office Consultation | | | | 99302 | SNF Initial Eval Level II | |
| | 99245 | Level V Office Consultation | | | | 99303 | SNF Initial Eval Level III | |
| | | Domiciliary Care | | | | 99311 | Subsequent SNF Level I | |
| | 99321 | Domiciliary Care I NP | | | | 99312 | Subsequent SNF Level II | |
| | 99322 | Domiciliary Care II NP | | | | 99313 | Subsequent SNF Level III | |
| | 99323 | Domiciliary Care III NP | | | | | Other Charges | |
| | 99331 | Domiciliary FU I | | | | 90005 | Failed Appointment | |
| | 99332 | Domiciliary FU II | | | | 90846 | Family without Patient Present | |
| | 99333 | Domiciliary FU III | | | | 90847 | Family with Patient Present | |

PLACE OF SERVICE ____OFFICE ____HOSPITAL ____EMERGENCY ROOM ____HOME ____SNF

Diagnosis Code:_____

Charges:_____    Payments:_____

Next Appointment _____

Jonathan M. Kersun, M.D.
PA LICENSE: MD051112-L    Tax ID:

FIGURE 4–1.    Example of a superbill.

## ∎ STATIONERY

You will need to purchase business cards, stationery, envelopes, statements, and practice-opening announcements. These items also can be purchased from a medical supply company (such as Histaccount, 800-645-5220).

## ∎ FURNITURE AND DÉCOR

Purchasing furniture and decorating the office can be a lot of fun. Here one gets to put one's own personal stamp on the establishment. The issue of how personalized a psychiatric office should be is often discussed in residency training. Personalization of an office can be considered in terms of the patient's comfort and your own tolerance for exposure—that is, for how revealing you want to be in terms of showing personal photos, diplomas, and memorabilia. There are no hard and fast rules in this regard except that it's a good idea to think about the matter. Your patients will notice the way your office is decorated and the way the furniture is arranged. It will be one of the many perceptions they have about you, and it will affect them and stimulate a response within them.

One study in the psychological literature looked at the effect of office décor and therapist gender on the perception of credibility (Bloom et al. 1977). Subjects were shown two different types of offices, the traditional professional office (desk between client and therapist, filing cabinet, diplomas on the wall) and the humanistic office (no desk between client and therapist, posters on the wall). Subjects were also told the gender of the therapist and then asked to form an impression of the doctor. Subjects consistently perceived the therapist as safer and more credible when a female therapist was in the traditional office and a male therapist was in the humanistic office. Thus, before ever meeting you, the patient is going to have perceptions about you based on what he or she sees. These perceptions will be influenced by the psychological makeup that the patient brings to the treatment situation.

The psychiatrist's office will have a psychological effect on the patient. For example, the office can be associated for a patient with meaningful experiences from the patient's life story. It can be interesting and sometimes helpful to the patient to explore his or her experience in this regard. One patient commented, "I like the way your office smells; it reminds me of my grandfather's house. I did not feel that my parents loved me, but I did feel my grandparents did."

From a practical standpoint, good advice is to treat the patient as if he or she were a guest in your own home. Coming to a psychiatric office can be difficult and anxiety producing; therefore, the more you can help a patient feel comfortable and at ease, the better. An office that is "medical" can have an overly sterile feel, not promoting sufficient warmth and comfort to facilitate the patient's opening up and sharing his or her inner life experience. On the other hand, overpersonalization—having a lot of personal effects on display—might focus too much attention on the doctor, generating discomfort in the other direction. One way to think about this issue is to contemplate the difference between displaying a photo of one's family as opposed to an art print that you happen to find attractive. The photo of your family is more directly personal than the art print in that it provides a more explicit view of your life. Displaying a photo of this sort may therefore have a seductive quality. An art print, on the other hand, is personal in that it reflects the interests and aesthetic preferences of the psychiatrist, from which the imaginative patient could deduce much. However, it is less explicit. It is also important to bear in mind that your patients will be seeing and experiencing the décor of the office. A lavishly decorated office could be uncomfortable for people of lower socioeconomic standing. Alternatively, an austerely decorated office might be uncomfortable for someone who is wealthy.

There is also the issue of hanging diplomas on the wall. Should you hang all diplomas, some diplomas, no diplomas, or just a medical license? Certainly, the convention is to display your credentials. Some doctors are proud of their educational achievements and like to display their diplomas as a sign of their accomplishments. Patients may assume that the pieces of paper confer qualification and ability. It is, of course, possible to practice without displaying any credentials at all. Although untraditional, this approach can be warm and personal. The patient then has to deal directly with the doctor; the patient can inquire about the doctor's credentials, and a discussion can ensue about what they mean.

None of the preceding discussion is meant to be taken as a literal "how to." It is merely intended to stimulate your thinking and give you some ideas to contemplate as you set up your office. Some patients are going to be curious and inquire about your décor; some will be curious and not inquire; and others will seem not to be at all curious. Any position that a patient might adopt is potentially valuable in terms of trying to understand him or her. Overall, when decorating the office, keep in mind the words "personal yet professional."

The waiting room is generally the first place a patient sees when coming to your office. It is nice for patients to be greeted with a pleasant, quiet, and peaceful space. A comfortable sofa and one or more comfortable chairs are usually necessary. One does not want to have only a sofa because this can put people into proximity that is uncomfortably close when more than one person is waiting. A coat rack and an umbrella stand are also good to have. A table with several magazines can provide a pleasant diversion for patients while they are waiting. Magazines that are light and easy to read are often most interesting to people in "waiting mode." One might have a magazine that is edited to be of interest to men (*Sports Illustrated, GQ, Men's Health*), a magazine that is edited to be of interest to women (*Self, Glamour, Cosmopolitan*), a magazine that is news oriented (*Newsweek, Time*), an entertainment magazine (*Entertainment Weekly, People*), and a travel magazine (*Travel and Leisure, Condé Nast Traveler*), and most people enjoy *Consumer Reports*. Magazines such as *The New Yorker, Harper's*, and *The New Republic*, while excellent and interesting magazines, are not easy to flip through. In general it is a good idea to put some thought into the choice of magazines in terms of finding reading that will be of some interest to people and might also reflect the doctor's tastes. There are a number of subscription services through which one can acquire magazines (such as EBSCO, 800-527-5901). Using a subscription service can be helpful because all of your magazines are renewed one time yearly and are paid for with one bill. Should you move offices, the subscription service will notify all of the magazines of the new address.

The lighting of the waiting room makes a significant difference in terms of the overall tone of the room. It is nice if the waiting room is softly lit, not lit by harsh overhead or fluorescent lighting. Soft lighting can be accomplished by using floor and table lamps. Having soft classical or jazz music playing can be comforting to people and can also provide somewhat of a sound barrier for nearby consultation rooms. You can also purchase a white noise generator (such as Marpac Sound Screen, 800-522-5969) to help keep sound from a nearby consultation room minimized.

Another nice touch in a waiting room is to have some plants or flowers. There are many different kinds of plants that do not require tremendous maintenance; some, such as a rubber plant, do not even need much light. There are also some very attractive artificial plants you can use that can cut down on upkeep and cost. Fresh flowers also can provide a lovely highlight to a waiting room. One of the authors has an established account with an area florist who delivers two bunches of fresh flowers every other week, one for the waiting room, one for the consultation room. The cost of $25 per delivery, or $50 per month, has been well worth it for all the pleasure that has come from fresh flowers brightening up the office.

# ▍ THE CONSULTATION ROOM

This is the space where you will ultimately spend a lot of time. It is to your advantage if you like this room. If you do not like your consultation room, you will feel a very subtle yet perceptible "drag." On the other hand, if you like your office space, being in it is a very pleasant experience and makes working with patients all the more enjoyable. It can be interesting to experience more than one office and notice the effect that a given space has on your mind. The amount of furniture you have in your office will, to a certain extent, be determined by the amount of space you have. A comfortable chair is certainly a priority. It is a good idea to consider investing some money in a chair that is ergonomically designed and fosters good posture; sitting in a chair that is overly soft can cause slouching, which can contribute to the development of back pain. Having at least one comfortable chair for patients is also necessary. Some prefer a couch for patients to sit on. Of course, for one pursuing analytic practice, a couch will be necessary. If the doctor and patient are sitting in chairs that are somewhat similar, a sense of equality is created. If the doctor is sitting on a large, overstuffed chair and the patient is sitting on a smaller chair, a sense of inequality and hierarchy might be induced that could be uncomfortable for the patient. You need to decide whether you want a desk in the office. It can be helpful to have a space on which to write and in which to store things. On the other hand, an office without a desk can have a more comfortable, living-room feel. Some psychiatrists have been able to fashion their offices in such a way that there are two doors into the consultation room, one for patients entering from the waiting room, one for exiting patients. This arrangement affords an increased level of privacy so that patients do not see one another. Often, however, it is not possible to configure your office in this way. You also need to decide how you are going to arrange the furniture in the office (Goldman and Stricker 1972; Hollender and Ford 1990). In general, it is best for the doctor and the patient to be sitting across from one another without a desk between them. The optimal distance between chairs is the usual conversational distance. Placing a desk between you and your patient can be off-putting and cold. Although some paranoid patients might do better with this arrangement, most patients prefer their doctor to be seated across from them without the barrier of a desk.

# ▐ OFFICE EQUIPMENT

A phone and a message recording system are necessities in starting a practice. You can either purchase a phone with an answering system built in or use a voice mail system established through the phone company. Both options work well, but phones with message recording systems tend to become less reliable and wear out over time. Some phone answering systems can be set up to forward calls to activate a pager. Some psychiatrists use a professional answering service. Such a service allows for a live voice to pick up your calls. The service will page you if the call is an emergency, or they will send you a faxed message for routine calls. In all, a professional answering service is probably an unnecessary expense when you are just starting out.

A fax machine is another important piece of equipment that you will need for faxing patient information and receiving lab data. You can have the fax machine run on a separate phone line, or you can use "identi-ring," a less expensive option. For this option, a separate phone number but not a separate line is established for the fax machine, thereby creating two numbers for one line. A different ring quality is assigned to each number; the phone is set to one ring quality, and the fax machine is set to pick up for the second ring quality. This phone company feature works quite well, the major limitation being that you cannot use the telephone when you are sending or receiving a fax. Early on, this limitation tends not to be very problematic because the use of the fax machine is often minimal.

You should also consider purchasing a photocopy machine. For an investment of several hundred dollars, this machine often comes in quite handy. If you are working with a billing company, you will need to copy and send the company billing and receivable information. In order to save money, you can decide to put off purchasing a photocopy machine as long as you have access to one nearby. Early on in practice, one of the authors went to a copying center on a weekly basis for photocopying, always being extremely careful to guard the privacy of patients.

## ▌ RECORDS

You will also need to establish a patient recordkeeping system. A relatively simple system involves having a manila folder for each patient. On the left-hand side of the open folder, you can place a medication record and documentation of patient allergies. On the right-hand side of the folder, you can keep laboratory data and notes and correspondence with primary or referring physicians. (It is both professionally courteous and a good patient care practice to send an initial letter after a consultation, second opinion, or referral.) Patient notes can be handwritten, dictated or typed on a small desktop word processor. The frequency and level of detail in patient notes is an individual decision; there is no definitive standard.

You will find that as your practice evolves, so too will your record keeping system. In the early stages, it is a good idea to have a complete and thorough record written in the standard medical fashion: CC, HPI, PpsyH, PMH, Meds, Social History, MSE, A/P (chief complaint, history of present illness, past psychiatric history, past medical history, medications, social history, mental status examination, assessment/plan). Your file should also contain written correspondence with the referring physician, other health care providers, or family members. It may be useful to keep a record of critical incidents or important conversations with family members. Some insurance companies, such as Medicare, require documentation. It is the right of the insurance company, should they desire, to audit your patient records for the purpose of verifying services rendered. Therefore, it is a good idea to acquaint yourself with the documentation requirements of the insurance companies with which you participate.

More and more psychiatrists are opting to use computers for their patient records. A number of software programs are available to facilitate this process, including some designed specifically for mental health practice (for example: MedWare, 800–819–5563, http://www.medware.com; Saner Software Inc., 630–513–5599; http://www.ShrinkRapt.com). One of the authors uses ShrinkRapt, a program that significantly enhances the efficiency of practice. Not only does software help you organize medical documentation, it also can simultaneously streamline scheduling and billing. The programs will usually help with bookkeeping; some will even facilitate insurance claim processing. If you are considering using a computer, contact a number of different companies and see which software is most appealing. Find out who has the best technical support. Ask the company for references, and call other psychiatrists who use the software to see how it works for them. (The use of computers in private practice is further discussed in Chapter 7 of this volume.)

# ▌ CONCLUSION

There is an elegant simplicity to psychiatric practice. At its essence, psychiatry involves two people sitting in a room participating in a shared endeavor to help one of the two participants—the patient—deal more effectively with the struggles of his or her mind. The details mentioned in this chapter are relevant to psychiatric practice, but they are not what the practice is all about. Your office will enhance and enable your success if it is conveniently located, comfortable, and well run. For the most part, patients should like coming to your office and find it a place where they are well cared for. You should also like your office and find it to be a place where you can work in a thoughtful, efficient, and effective manner.

# ■ REFERENCES

Bloom LJ, Weigel RG, Trautt GM: "Therapeugenic" factors in psychotherapy: effects of office décor and subject-therapist sex pairing on the perception of credibility. J Consult Clin Psychol 45:867–73, 1977

Goldman GD, Stricker G (ed): Practical Problems of a Private Psychotherapy Practice. Springfield, IL, Charles C Thomas, 1972

Hollender MH, Ford CV: Dynamic Psychotherapy: An Introductory Approach. Washington, DC, American Psychiatric Press, 1990

# 5

# MARKETING PRIVATE PRACTICE PSYCHIATRY

## Ten Internal and Ten External Practice Tips

*Marcia L. Brauchler, M.P.H., CPHQ, CPC*

Building any practice takes hard work, but marketing a psychiatric practice poses many unique challenges. Relying on patient referrals is tricky because of privacy concerns. Building a referral base can be difficult because of established managed behavioral health care organization (MBHO) referral patterns—which may comfortably be directing business to existing groups—and also because of network participation requirements, which may delay new-provider participation for months while verifying credentials. Also, for many providers, there may be a stigma associated with advertising directly to patients. Despite these challenges, don't give up. The ability to successfully market your services will directly affect your practice's

For their contributions, special thanks to Paul Angotti, Manager, Management Design, LLC, Colorado Springs, CO; Laura Lemon, M.B.A., Primary Care Liaison for The Medical Center of Aurora, Parker, CO; Michele Silverman, M.A., San Clemente, CA; and Lara Sanders, Marketing Consultant, Lakewood, CO.

bottom line. In this chapter I present several marketing techniques—both internal and external—to help you build a successful psychiatric practice.

Efficient and effective operation of the practice is a prerequisite to marketing. Without good operations, much of the marketing effort and expense will be entirely wasted. For example, if a patient tries to call in response to being handed a business card for your practice but can't get through on the phone line, the marketing effort was a waste. Here are some tips for the internal operations of your practice that affect marketing.

## ∎ TEN TIPS TO INTERNAL OPERATIONS FOR MARKETING

### #1: Treat Every Patient the Way You Would Like To Be Treated as a Patient

This first tip for your practice is a variation of the Golden Rule. Think back to your last physician visit as a patient. What do you remember about the visit? If your first memory is of an overwhelming amount of paperwork during your check-in, do your best to minimize that for your patients. For example, your office could send the paperwork to the patient when he or she phones to schedule the first appointment. In addition to the necessary insurance and registration forms, this information could include details on your practice. If you remember being impressed by the driving directions and parking instructions you received in the mail before your first appointment with a new physician, you can implement a similar program for your practice's new patients.

### #2: Establish Clinically Appropriate Protocols for Contacting Existing Patients

Protocols should be defined by age and sex, medical history, managed care plan requirements, clinical norms, and most important, patient requests. When a patient schedules a follow-up appointment, consider asking the patient in advance if a reminder phone call the day before is permissible. If so, ask specifically which telephone number is appropriate to call and how much information is appropriate to leave in the message. *Retaining your existing patients for already-scheduled appointments is one of the most critical aspects of internal marketing.* If a patient's therapy would be optimized by meeting with you again after a specific period of time, for example in 2 weeks or 6 months after medication is discontinued, be sure to have a system in place for you and your office staff to initiate a recall to the patient. Also, using the data on existing patients, such as diagnoses, you can proactively contact patients. New medical information may be of interest, such as a new medication being advertised on television or in magazines that may provide a reason to suggest that the patient schedule an appointment.

## #3: Be Proactive in Solving Problems With Patients

When a situation arises, do not ignore it, even if the practice is not responsible for the problem. For example, if an outside billing company charged the patient a balance that was later reimbursed by insurance coverage, the patient may never fully understand the situation unless someone contacts her to hear her view of the situation, communicate the practice's point of view, and offer some sort of acceptable reconciliation. Similar contact should take place for a scheduling misunderstanding (for example, if the patient shows up for an appointment on the wrong day and cannot be worked in) and for other patient inconveniences, regardless of fault.

## #4: Provide a Complete Line of Psychiatric Services

Providing a full range of services can dissuade existing patients from approaching another physician in the same specialty who has a different practice emphasis or reputation. Types of services may include individual therapy, marriage and family therapy, group therapy, employee assistance program (EAP) services, bilingual/bicultural capability, psychological testing, and crisis intervention. Other specialty niches include adolescent substance abuse, parent training, family skills training, eye movement desensitization and reprocessing (EMDR), grief and bereavement, premarital counseling, alcohol abuse treatment, stress management, pain management, chronic illness, and geriatric care. If you refer a patient out of the practice to another practitioner with a specialization that you do not offer, consider cross-referrals. When contacting a physician to whom you are referring a client, notify the physician of your intent to refer patients with specific needs to him or her. Take the opportunity to inform the physician about the specialization of your practice, and ask for the courtesy of receiving referrals as well.

## #5: Communicate Services to Patients Through Videos or CD-ROM

Videos can be used in the reception area or in exam rooms, or they can be given to patients to take home. The video content can be entirely customized by your practice through the help of a graphic design or media marketing firm. The content can include your practice philosophy, credentials, and specific services offered. Perhaps patient testimonials could be used as external references of your services. With less expense and production time, a CD-ROM could be made and distributed to patients with the same information in a written format or on electronic presentation slides. These media allow the patient to review your marketing material in greater depth while in the privacy of his or her home, or perhaps to share the materials with other interested family members or contacts.

## #6: Use Any Reasonable Excuse to Make Announcements to Patients

Announcing news to patients will keep your practice present in their minds. Announce the addition of a new practitioner to the practice, new equipment, new training and certifications of the practitioners and staff, or new office hours. Forms of announcements include posting in the reception area, fliers inserted with the patient billing statements, newspaper advertisements, and postcards or letters sent to patients directly. These continual friendly reminders about your practice may prompt a patient to call and schedule an appointment that otherwise might have been thought about but not acted on.

## #7: Publish Your Fee Schedule and Any Payment Plans

Offer discounts for cash-paying patients who pay at the time of service. The savings associated with generating statements and mailing them after the service can be passed along to the patient, and you receive the payment immediately. One caution: avoid sending numerous repeat bills and/or "this is not a bill" statements. This inefficient billing practice may be based on keeping the patient in the loop about insurance payments, but it generally serves only to confuse and annoy patients. In a similar vein, instruct your billing company to write off small balances, for example less than $1.00, to not send patient notices for negligent amounts that are less than the cost of postage. These patient invoices cause more trouble than they are worth, and do not generate goodwill with your patients.

## #8: Document Patient Satisfaction and Incorporate High Scores Into Your Marketing Efforts

You may want to include your satisfaction rating in mailings to referral sources to make them even more comfortable with sending patients to you.

A sample patient satisfaction survey is included for use with your existing patients (Appendix 5–A). You may want to consider having a box in your waiting room so that patients can return the surveys before they leave, for their convenience and for immediate feedback. To increase the likelihood of a response if they leave with the survey, include your fax number and/or your mailing address on the survey. If you can incorporate, for example, a 95% patient satisfaction with their treatment or 98% satisfaction with ease of scheduling an appointment into your marketing materials, these statistics promote positive associations with your office to current and future patients.

### #9: Consider Mailing a Mental Health Newsletter

A newsletter for patients can include medical articles and tips for improving psychological health. With proper citations to the original source, putting this together this can be as easy as summarizing some of the current medical literature in your specialty, and it is another way to remind patients about your practice while conveying timely medical insights.

### #10: Have an Inviting, Homelike Waiting Room and Restroom

The homelike qualities can be attained through the addition of plants, cozy chairs, and soft lighting. You want your office to be a comfortable, well-kept place for clients. Strive to create a refuge from your patients' busy, fast-paced schedules.

## ▮ TEN TIPS FOR EXTERNAL MARKETING

### #1: Choose the Right Location

Identifying where to locate your private practice is the most important decision you can make when starting on your own. Hire a consulting firm that specializes in performing market surveys, or piece together a survey on your own. Start with the provider directories from MBHOs to get an idea of how many psychiatrists are in your vicinity and any relevant specializations. Provider directories from medical insurance plans will give you contact information for potential referring physicians and hospitals. Check the yellow pages in the phone book for information on other practicing physicians. Use the hospital medical staff roster for more information on what services are available and where they are located. When starting a practice in a competitive market, consider client convenience; you may wish to offer after-work hours and weekend appointments. Your best marketing expenses, initially, will be placing an advertisement in the phone book (even just the practice name and phone number) and printing business cards.

## #2: Develop an Informational Brochure About You and Your Practice

The brochure will promote the practice and reduce the need for phone calls to the office for basic information such as office hours or your mailing address. Consider including your practice's policies on appointment cancellations and payment-for-services in the brochure. The brochure and an associated packet of introductory materials can be sent to a patient in advance of the first visit. There are many benefits from investing in brochures. Patient brochures do not have to be prohibitively expensive to create. They can be distributed to patients in a variety of ways. Brochures can be mailed to new patients when appointments are made well in advance, and they can be mailed to people who move into the community. They can be given to patients in the office at the end of the visit with a statement like, "This brochure will help you understand how we can work together effectively to provide the best quality care. Please read it and call if you have any questions." Stacks of brochures should be left in the reception area, provided to referring practitioners to give to patients being referred, and made available at speaking engagements, health fairs, and any other promotional forums. Physicians should carry their business cards or brochures with them to give to a prospective patient or referral source. Appendix 5–B offers an outline to get you started on developing your practice brochure.

## #3: Market Directly to Your Referral Sources

Use any reasonable excuse to contact referral sources, including other psychiatrists and behavioral health practitioners, primary care physicians, and even MBHOs. Such contacts generally fall into two categories: announcements and medical information. Announce the addition of a new practitioner to the practice, new services, or new hours. Medical information, especially information that may help the referring practitioners take good care of patients and know when it is appropriate to refer a patient, can be looked at as a professional courtesy in addition to providing a reason to contact a referral source. You may want to consider sending surveys regularly to all providers that referred patients to you, letting them know that you care about their experience when interacting with your practice. A sample survey is provided (Appendix 5–C).

## #4: Always Respect Your Referral Sources

When you receive a referral from another practitioner, provide only the care requested by the referring practitioner and indicated by medical necessity for the patient's condition. Return the patient to the referring practitioner for all care that is within the practitioner's capability. As soon as possible after seeing a patient sent from a referral source, send the source a complete report. Reports should be sent within 24 hours of seeing the patient unless test results are pending. Reports should include findings, your treatment plan, recommendations for treatment by the referring practitioner, and the scheduled follow-up date, if any. There is no need to include sensitive patient information. Consider asking the patient if he or she would like to see a copy of the letter being sent to the referring provider. The best expression of appreciation for a referral is a prompt, complete report rather than a thank-you letter or card.

Keep in mind also that when a referred patient does not show up for an appointment (or does not make one), it is important to report this to the referring practitioner. Otherwise, the practitioner generally will assume that the patient was seen but the consulting doctor just did not bother to send a report.

## #5: Welcome Your Colleagues in Medicine Who Are New to Practice or New to the Area

When a new practitioner of any medical specialty sets up practice or joins a practice, initiate contact, welcome him or her, and offer help with getting started. The effort will be so welcome and so unusual that the new practitioner will be inclined to refer patients to you first.

## #6: Understand the Insurance Carrier or Payer Landscape in Your Marketplace

The Division of Insurance (or other government entity in your state with oversight responsibility for insurance carriers) has information that is publicly available on licensed MBHOs in your state and county as well as the number of insured individuals. The government agency Web site or publication will give you an idea of which payers represent the bulk of the business and may be worthwhile participation networks to pursue. Learn which medical insurance companies require referrals from primary care physicians. For EAPs, consider introducing yourself to the larger employers' human resources staff. When employees are seeking particular mental health services, they may ask for referrals from the human resources contact, who would then feel comfortable passing along your practice information. In the effort to stay on the best insurance panels and networks, proactive marketing to carriers is effective. For this reason, consider communicating new services, additional capability, or cost-savings techniques to major insurance carriers. You may also volunteer to sit on the MBHO or medical insurance company administrative committees, such as pharmacy and therapeutics, utilization management, credentialing, risk management, and quality management. Most companies pay practitioners small stipends for meeting attendance. Meetings generally occur quarterly over dinner and last a few hours. To volunteer, contact the health plan's provider relations department.

## #7: Train Your Billing Staff or Outsourced Billing Company in Your Policies and Procedures

In an effort to collect all the fees the physicians have earned, the billing staff is often in an adversarial role with carriers and patients. If the staff is too aggressive in collecting, carriers may remove the physician from their network and patients may go elsewhere. Your billing staff should be advised to follow the Golden Rule (see internal marketing tip #1) when dealing with patients. To minimize the possibility of alienating insurance companies, your billing staff should strive to establish a positive and professional working relationship with the practice's major insurance carriers. Billing staff should visit the carrier's offices to meet the people who process claims or authorizations and should have regular meetings at your office with the health plans' provider relations representatives. You will find that making the effort to establish positive working relationships expedites problem solving and leads to more referrals to your practice.

## #8: To Find Self-Pay Patients, Get Involved in Your Community

Any topic related to current events or changes in treatments or techniques may provide a chance to educate the public through speaking opportunities. National Mental Health Day (or a similar event) may provide a good opening to seek speaking opportunities at community events or for church groups. Service clubs with weekly meetings may be the perfect place for you to present a program on psychiatric-related topics of interest. Although talk of this sort cannot be an overt push for patients, it provides an outstanding opportunity for you to showcase your treatment philosophy, personality, and professional expertise. This may attract patients or lead to referrals.

Contact local hospitals about presenting a continuing education program. Through contacting the medical staff department (or other administrative department in charge of arranging for continuing medical education credits), you may line up a speaking opportunity to address referring physicians. You may also receive an honorarium for your presentation.

Although slightly more difficult to arrange, public television and radio appearances are also excellent opportunities to establish yourself as an expert on a topic that may attract patients to your practice. Keep in mind when promoting yourself to television and radio stations that they are generally more interested in topics that are sensational or timely.

If there is a large employer in your area, you may approach the human resources director or other company executive to offer topics that would be in line with their employee assistance program, such as stress management or effective treatments of depression or conflict resolution. Consider approaching a local community college or other educational institution to teach a one-day course or workshop for students or the general public.

## #9: Advertising Can Be Subtle

A press release to newspapers, radio, or television can be successful—and it is essentially free advertising. Rather than buy advertising space, the practice can send press releases or pitch story ideas for radio and television or write columns or editorials for the newspaper. The press release or story pitch must be newsworthy and provide some information that the general public cares about and does not already know. This is a broad form of marketing that targets the general public and may result in referrals to the practice once you are seen as an expert on the subject in the media. Sample formats for a press release and a pitch to the media for a topic on which you can be used as an expert are provided (Appendix 5–D and Appendix 5–E).

## #10: Each Time You Meet Someone New, It Is an Opportunity to Network and Promote Your Practice

Like any independent business owner, you are expected to be your own best marketing representative. Networking with your referral sources might be the easiest. Keep in mind the principle of quid pro quo when you are networking. Buy your contact a cup of coffee or treat him or her to lunch. In exchange for the person's time, do not hesitate to share ideas on business practices, marketing ideas that you are thinking of undertaking, and the possibility of co-promoting your businesses. The directories and materials you gathered for understanding your marketplace and where to start a practice (see external tip #1) may come in handy again. If you don't yet have established referral sources, use a directory from the local hospital or a large health plan in your market to identify the names, specialties, and locations of surrounding physicians, emergency rooms, and psychiatric hospitals, and contact those offices to inquire about their current referral patterns and the strength of those relationships. You may want to ask these providers about health plans that cover a large part of their patient populations so that you can also participate with those insurance networks and be available for referrals.

## ∎ CONCLUSION

Marketing additional visits to existing patients already in the practice is the simplest marketing process. There is very little cost and effort required to retain patients and provide additional services to them. Therefore, direct your first marketing effort toward current patients.

Create a plan for marketing your services and work with others to brainstorm creative ideas for promoting your practice. Try to incorporate ideas from both the internal and external marketing tips in this chapter, but by no means are these lists exhaustive. After identifying your specific goal, create a timeline to accomplish each step effectively. Stick to a plan for accomplishing your marketing over time—a successful practice is not built overnight. Set goals. For example, try to make four networking contacts a month and plan to complete a patient brochure within the first month of establishing your practice. Include time to evaluate the success of your efforts. Incorporate your successes into future marketing. If you receive 30 completed patient surveys in your first quarter of practice, incorporate the positive statistics into the letter you send to referring physicians, or create a summary of the statistics for a poster in your waiting room. Marketing is an investment in your practice, with returns in the form of more patients or better reimbursement for patients realized over the life of your practice.

## APPENDIX 5–A

# Sample Patient Survey Questionnaire

## [PRACTICE NAME]

## PATIENT SURVEY QUESTIONNAIRE

## [address, phone and fax number]

We want to provide the best possible medical care in a way that is as comfortable and convenient to patients as possible. To accomplish this, we need your feedback. Please take a moment to complete this questionnaire, letting us know what we are doing right and how we can improve.

All responses will be kept strictly confidential. Feel free to add comments in the blank spaces as necessary.

| **BEFORE YOUR OFFICE VISIT:** (If no, please explain) | YES | NO |
|---|---|---|
| 1. Was the person scheduling your appointment friendly? | ☐ | ☐ |
| 2. Did you have trouble getting an appointment at a time you desired? | ☐ | ☐ |
| 3. Was the staff helpful in finding appointment times to satisfy your needs? | ☐ | ☐ |
| 4. Are your phone calls handled in a prompt, courteous manner? | ☐ | ☐ |
| 5. Have you ever called our doctors? If yes, was your call returned promptly? | ☐ | ☐ |
| 6. Was your call to the doctor during normal business hours? | ☐ | ☐ |
| 7. Do you mind if a staff member responds to some of your calls? | ☐ | ☐ |
| 8. Is the location of our office convenient for you? | ☐ | ☐ |
| 9. Are the office hours convenient for you? | ☐ | ☐ |
| 10. Is ample parking available for you? | ☐ | ☐ |

## AT THE TIME OF YOUR VISIT
**(If no, please explain)**                                  **YES**    **NO**

1. Is our waiting area comfortable?                            ☐        ☐

2. Do you feel that the reception and consulting room areas
   were clean and well-kept?                                   ☐        ☐

3. Was our front office personnel friendly and courteous?     ☐        ☐

4. Was the registration process quick and efficient?          ☐        ☐

5. Was your wait too long in the reception area before
   seeing the doctor?                                          ☐        ☐

6. Do you find the doctor friendly and courteous?             ☐        ☐

7. Do you feel the doctor is interested in you as a person?   ☐        ☐

8. Do you feel the doctor spends enough time with you?        ☐        ☐

9. If you received a prescription, did you receive adequate
   instructions regarding medications and follow-up care?     ☐        ☐

10. Was the arrangement of follow-up visits convenient?       ☐        ☐

## AFTER YOUR VISIT
**(If no, please explain)**

                                                             **YES**    **NO**
1. Do you feel that the outcome of your medical care
   was adequate?                                               ☐        ☐

2. Do you feel that any test results were obtained promptly?  ☐        ☐

3. Do you feel you had the opportunity to get questions
   answered during and/or after your visit?                   ☐        ☐

4. Do you feel that your bill was handled in an appropriate
   manner by the cashier?                                      ☐        ☐

5. Do you feel that your bill was accurate?                    ☐        ☐

6. Do you feel that your billing questions were adequately answered? ☐ ☐

7. Do you feel that our fees are reasonable? ☐ ☐

8. Are you satisfied enough with the care you received to recommend this practice to your family and/or friends? ☐ ☐

9. What most impressed you about our office and/or staff? ☐ ☐

10. How could we improve our service to you and your family? ☐ ☐

## BUSINESS OFFICE
**(If no, please explain)**

| | YES | NO |
|---|---|---|

1. Do you find our business personnel (practice manager, bookkeeper, etc.) friendly and courteous? ☐ ☐

2. Have you received a copy of our business policies? ☐ ☐

3. Have our payment and billing policies been explained to your satisfaction? ☐ ☐

4. Are you receiving adequate help with your insurance? ☐ ☐

### THANK YOU!
(include instructions on how to return)

## APPENDIX 5–B

# Suggested Outline for a Patient Brochure

The main objectives of a patient brochure are to educate patients and help the practice operate efficiently and effectively by

- Providing information about the practice and the practitioners
- Minimizing patient phone calls for basic information
- Collecting the patient portion of charges efficiently

Brochures should be left in the reception area and at the registration desk. In addition, a supply of brochures in the patient room(s) will allow practitioners and assistants to hand one to a patient when providing instructions, pointing to the relevant section of the brochure for emphasis. For example, when giving a new patient a prescription, the physician could hand the patient a brochure and point out the procedure for calling the pharmacy rather than the practice for a refill.

In addition, brochures can be mailed to new patients (with a welcome letter) so that the patient can read the practice policies and use the location map on the brochure to easily locate the office and know where to park.

Depending on the amount of information you plan to present, the brochure could be printed on 8½ x 11" paper and folded into thirds. A representative at your local copy shop can recommend paper stock and layout options. Because the brochure should be easy to read, use simple language with short sentences and paragraphs. Use a type size of 12 points or larger and try not to use more than two different fonts. The design of the brochure should project a consistent image by coordinating with the practice's stationery and even with the office decor.

The following list provides information that is generally included in a patient brochure:

1. Specialty interest and type of practice. Include, when appropriate:
   a. Solo or group practice
   b. Subspecialty
   c. Geographic area served
   d. Hospital affiliation

2. Physician information and personnel. Include, when appropriate:
   a. Degrees
   b. Residency programs
   c. Nonphysician staff of significance
   d. Special treatment techniques and/or equipment
   e. Photos, if available

3. Practice philosophy and/or practice motto or mission statement.

4. Information on appointments, such as cancellation policies, guidelines for walk-ins and work-ins, and office hours.

5. Contact information, including, as appropriate: main telephone number, mailing address, prescription refill telephone number, fax number, e-mail addresses, Web site address.

6. Financial policies: fees, billing, and collections. List of contracted insurance companies.

7. Statement on confidentiality of patient information.

8. Location map. Consider both a word description and a map.

9. Details on parking, if not obvious, including, as appropriate, availability and cost of metered street parking and valet parking, as well as a suggested allotment of time for parking and finding the office if this is likely to be a factor in a patient's timely arrival.

## APPENDIX 5–C

# Sample Referring Physician Questionnaire

**REFERRAL PRACTICE SURVEY**

Because we strive to provide the best possible medical care for our mutual patients, we would appreciate your help. Please complete this survey of your experience with us and your patients' opinions about our practice. All responses will be kept strictly confidential.

Please feel free to elaborate by way of an attachment to this survey, a telephone call, or a meeting—we really want to know what we are doing well and, when necessary, how we can serve you and your patients better. Thank you!

This response is from the office of Doctor _____

**A. Questions about our staff:**

1. Do you make appointments with our practice for your patients? ☐ Yes ☐ No
(If no, please skip to Part B.)

When you call for an appointment:

|  | Low | Medium | | High | |
|---|---|---|---|---|---|
|  | 1 | 2 | 3 | 4 | 5 |
| 2. Are you treated with courtesy? | ☐ | ☐ | ☐ | ☐ | ☐ |
| 3. Are timely appointments available? | ☐ | ☐ | ☐ | ☐ | ☐ |
| 4. Is our staff knowledgeable about insurance? | ☐ | ☐ | ☐ | ☐ | ☐ |
| 5. Is our staff clinically knowledgeable? | ☐ | ☐ | ☐ | ☐ | ☐ |

**B. Insurance and clinical information:**

| | | | | | |
|---|---|---|---|---|---|
| 1. Does your office receive all necessary information related to treatment? | ☐ | ☐ | ☐ | ☐ | ☐ |
| 2. Does your office receive requested information on time? | ☐ | ☐ | ☐ | ☐ | ☐ |

**C. Questions about the physician:**

1. With which physician(s) do you usually work?

_____

_____

| | Low | | Medium | | High |
|---|---|---|---|---|---|
| | 1 | 2 | 3 | 4 | 5 |
| 2. Are patients returned to your practice for services that you can provide? | ☐ | ☐ | ☐ | ☐ | ☐ |
| 3. Do you receive complete information about our findings, our plan of treatment, recommendations for your treatment, and when the patient should return to us? | ☐ | ☐ | ☐ | ☐ | ☐ |
| 4. Do you have enough information on our practice to give to referred patients? | ☐ | ☐ | ☐ | ☐ | ☐ |

## D. What do your patients tell you about our practice and physicians?

(When possible, please address specific appointments, treatment by the staff and physicians, communication with regard to treatment, charges, and insurance.)

_____

_____

_____

_____

_____

_____

## E. What suggestions do you have for us to improve our working relationship?

_____

_____

_____

_Thank you for your input._

## APPENDIX 5–D

# Sample Press Release

For Immediate Release

Contact: _____

(XXX) XXX-XXXX

**Dr. _____ _____ Opens New
Mental Health Practice Serving _____**

CITY, State—(Date), 2004— Dr. _____ _____ has announced the grand opening of his new practice, _____ to serve the mental health needs of _____(area), and will celebrate with an open house on _____ from ____ to ____.

_____ attended _____ medical school in _____, _____, and completed his residency at _____ and his psychiatric training/fellowship at _____, where he worked with _____.

_____ specializes in _____. The open house is your chance to meet with Dr. _____ and his staff. Refreshments will be served and from ____ to ____. Dr. _____ will present a short seminar on _____.

For more information about Dr. _____ and _____, please call (XXX) XXX-XXX or visit his Web site at www.mdmdmd.com.

## APPENDIX 5–E

# Sample Pitch to the Media for a Story in Which You Could Be Used as an Expert

### Local Psychiatrist, Dr. \_\_\_\_\_ _____, Offers Seminar on Overcoming Holiday Stress

- A significant percentage of the population in the United States admits to feeling increased levels of anxiety from October through January.

- Having coping mechanisms available can help individuals recognize the sources of stress and find ways to enjoy the holidays with friends and family.

- Dr. \_\_\_\_ offers new and interesting techniques for battling holiday stress, including: (describe)

# 6

# OBTAINING REIMBURSEMENT FOR OUTPATIENT SERVICES FROM MANAGED AND UNMANAGED INSURANCE

## Principles and Procedures

*Michael I. Bennett, M.D.*

Obtaining reimbursement for outpatient services from managed and un-managed insurance has become increasingly complex as insurers invent an ever-growing number of unique insurance products and methods that rely on clinical information to "manage the benefit." Obtaining reimbursement is a continual manifestation of Murphy's Law: Everything that can go wrong will go wrong. So, the following is a set of principles and procedures for combating the chaos and confusion that threaten to block payment for services rendered.

There are few clinicians of middle age or older who will not confess to nostalgia for the good old days when insurance played a small role in funding outpatient treatment and when insurance benefits, when available, were easily accessed by completing a one-page claim form, then billing the patient for the remaining balance after insurance had paid. Many clinicians today, after facing a mountain of rejected claims, refuse to take insurance and require their patients to pay their entire fee out of pocket or go elsewhere. There is no denying that the current system wastes time, imposes huge overhead costs on clinicians, and often results in unfair and frustrating payment denials. However, we cannot reject the current system without also refusing to treat a large segment of our community and disqualifying ourselves from an important part of our mission and our source of professional satisfaction. This chapter's goal is to help clinicians make the best of a complex insurance reimbursement system by learning how to avoid its pitfalls and make it pay what it should as often as possible. The basic principles and procedures are the same whether you use a billing agency to submit claims and track payments and paperwork or do it yourself.

## ∎ PRINCIPLES

### #1: Forge a Partnership With Your Patients
### Regarding Management of Their Insurance Resource

Patients need to understand that their insurance benefit has limits and that they will need to pay a portion of your fees. You need to educate them about the technical limits of their insurance benefit, the clinical factors that influence how much reimbursement their benefit will provide, and the methods you can and cannot use to help them get the most out of it. For instance, you might say:

> "I can help you make the most out of your insurance, but first I need to know how much and what type of coverage it provides for mental health treatment. Each insurance product is unique, and some provide less or no coverage for mental health problems, for the initial phase of treatment, or for treatment of problems other than severe mental illness. We need to know whether your insurance is 'managed,' that is, whether we must periodically provide your insurer with information about your treatment proving that it is 'medically necessary,' before they will 'authorize,'—guarantee—payment. *Medically necessary* means that a treatment is the least costly way of treating problems covered by your insurance benefit while meeting standards for effectiveness and safety. We also need to know whether your insurer recognizes me as a 'network provider,' a relationship that obliges them to pay me and may oblige me to accept a discounted fee."

## #2: Develop Procedures for Preventing Technical Problems From Blocking Claims Payment

The longer a claim goes unpaid, the more likely it is that an insurer will refuse to pay it, citing a policy for rejecting overdue claims or authorizations (for instance, more than 90 and 30 days, respectively, after services were performed). Insurance clerks are seldom empowered to waive claims rejections without your having to file an appeal in writing—a procedure that is, of course, likely to take as much time as the service itself. The best remedy is prevention.

## #3: For Managed Benefits, Determine Medical Necessity Without Regard to Insurers

As noted under Principle #1 above, managed insurance covers that part of treatment that is "medically necessary," that is, the least costly treatment that meets standards for safety and effectiveness, assuming that the treated problem is contractually covered. If you recommend treatment over and above this minimum, your patient may bear the cost. Misleading the insurer will ultimately jeopardize your credibility, making it harder for you to obtain authorization for the services to which your patients are entitled. Make your own determination of what is medically necessary; then you will be best prepared to advocate for your patient with the insurer. Procedures for determining medical necessity are described below in Procedure #2 in the "Medical Necessity" section.

An example: you and your patient believe he would do best with weekly psychotherapy for at least 6 months because he seems to respond positively to treatment and feels greatly helped with his problems, which include dysthymia but no major disability. You believe, however, that less frequent sessions would be almost as good because he works on his problems between sessions and does not appear likely to relapse when he misses one. You decide that every other week will probably be good enough for now, and less frequent sessions will be acceptable in the near future. You explain your reasoning and its purpose and propose to reconsider the intensity of his treatment frequently, using his input and what you observe to decide what is medically necessary.

## #4: Help Patients Anticipate Their Costs

A good evaluation can help patients anticipate and manage their costs, which are, as always, a potentially dangerous side effect of treatment. For instance, you might say:

"I believe your insurance will cover every-other-week treatment for the next 6 months because you have a 'parity diagnosis,' meaning that your symptoms qualify for a diagnosis of mental illness and this enhances your coverage. In addition, your history of self-harm and current experience of suicidal ideation put you in a high-risk category that also increases your entitlement. Including your co-pay of $20, treatment for the next 6 months would cost you less than $300."

# ∎ PROCEDURES

## #1: Set Up a Billing and Accounting System

You have four options for filing claims and keeping accounts: paper, a home computer with billing software, a professional computerized billing system, and a billing service. Table 6–1 summarizes the advantages and drawbacks of each.

### Paper: Tried and True, but an Endangered Species?

If you have no more than a few patients at a time, it is easy to keep your accounts and fill in forms by paper. Paper requires no programming and cannot crash. After you fill in a patient's first claim form, you can use a copier to avoid most data entry on the rest. And because mailing paper claims is not considered electronics claims submission (ECS), their use may exempt you from federal Health Insurance Portability and Accountability Act (HIPAA) requirements. On the other hand, paper claims may soon be prohibited.

### The Home Computer

If you have a large practice and like to play with a computer (meaning that you enjoy turning on a computer and then figuring out something useful to do with it), then there is well-established management software to help you with recordkeeping. It costs no more than $500 and can be used to fill out claims, keep your accounts and, if you like, keep clinical notes, without necessarily requiring ECS and thus HIPAA compliance. Producing and mailing claims for 200 patients for a month of services should take you no more than 2 hours, including stuffing and stamping envelopes. Although such a system usually saves time by speeding data entry, reducing arithmetical errors, and churning out claims forms, it can, on occasion, consume huge amounts of time in the way that computers do when a disk drive crashes or a new operating system conflicts with older software or hardware. If you choose management software, remember that reliability is far more important than an attractive interface or an additional option. Select long-established software with a large user base and well supported by a prosperous company. Also, you must back up your data religiously. Low-cost practice-management software, in particular, is prone to crash. (Computing options are discussed more fully in Chapter 7 of this volume.)

### Professional Billing Systems

If you operate a large office, you may opt for billing software designed for large medical practices and supported by larger companies.

### Billing Services

For many clinicians with large practices, a billing service is easier than doing your own bills. There is a small fee for each claim submitted, and you must comply with HIPAA regulations because your claims are being submitted electronically. Your time for data collecting and processing is no less than it would be for other methods because you must provide the same information to the billing service that you would otherwise gather for your own system. But a billing service protects you from the vagaries of computer crashes and spares you from generating, stuffing, stamping, and mailing claims and patient bills. Using ECS, it obtains an immediate response from insurers that identifies problems of ineligibility or missing authorizations before they can invalidate a claim by causing excessive delay. More important, it deals with the 5% of denied claims that consume 95% of your time: the lost claims, missing authorizations, expired policies, and other manifestations of Murphy's Law that would otherwise force you to navigate long telephone menus and listen to bad music while "our agents are busy serving other customers."

Appendix 6–A is a sample outpatient claims form, the standard HCFA 1500, filled in using the standard format that almost all insurers (other than Medicare) require. For most insurers, the only areas of variability are Box 23, in which some insurers require you to place an authorization number, and Box 33, in which you may be required to put the provider number by which that insurer identifies you. Medicare's unique requirements, which changed as recently as a month prior to this writing, are displayed in Appendix 6–B. The forms are available from any medical stationery supplier.

## #2: Ask Prospective Patients to Obtain Insurance Information

Ask prospective patients to gather information from their insurer that will help you bill efficiently and adjust your treatment plan to the realities of their coverage.

**TABLE 6–1.** Advantages and disadvantages of different billing systems

| Advantages | Disadvantages |
| --- | --- |
| **Paper-based methods** | |
| • Simple, predictable, crashproof.<br>• Low cost for startup and maintenance.<br>• Simple tricks, such as copying claims forms after one-time entry of demographic data, can save considerable time. | • One must often enter data twice (on a claim and in a ledger).<br>• Arithmetic must be done on a calculator.<br>• Each claim form or patient bill requires some work by hand.<br>• Ledgers can be damaged or lost, are not easily duplicated, and take up increasing amounts of filing space.<br>• Pursuing denied claims and missing payments is time-consuming.<br>• Paper claims may soon be prohibited. |
| **Computer-based systems** | |
| • Data are entered once only.<br>• Calculations are automatic and accurate.<br>• Produces claims and patient bills rapidly, ready for mailing, and in printed form rather than hand written.<br>• Alerts may remind you when authorizations are due or payments are missing. | • Computer crashes can be dreadful.<br>• Startup costs of hardware and software are about $1,500.<br>• System needs updating to respond to changing data requirements and periodic obsolescence of all computer systems.<br>• Pursuing denied claims and missing payments is time-consuming.<br>• Unless software is flexible and/or well supported, it may be unable to meet unique requirements for each insurer. |
| **Professional billing systems** | |
| • Data are entered once only.<br>• Calculations are automatic and accurate.<br>• Produces claims and patient bills rapidly, ready for mailing, and in printed form rather than hand written; or may do electronic claims submission.<br>• Alerts may remind you when authorizations are due or payments are missing.<br>• Electronic claims submission identifies problems at once and speeds payments. | • Computer crashes can be dreadful.<br>• Startup costs of hardware and software are about $2,500.<br>• System needs updating to respond to changing data requirements and periodic obsolescence of all computer systems.<br>• Pursuing denied claims and missing payments is time-consuming.<br>• Electronic claims submission requires your office to comply with HIPAA regulations. |

TABLE 6–1. Advantages and disadvantages of different billing systems *(continued)*

| Advantages | Disadvantages |
| --- | --- |
| **Billing services** | |
| • Data are entered once only.<br>• Calculations are automatic and accurate.<br>• Produces claims and patient bills rapidly, ready for mailing, and in print form rather than hand written; or may do electronic claims submission.<br>• Alerts may remind you when authorizations are due or payments are missing.<br>• Electronic claims submission identifies problems at once and speeds payments.<br>• Service staff can correct most claims denials. | • Cost per claim may be more than for a do-it-yourself system if you do a large number of claims.<br>• Electronic claims submission requires your office to comply with HIPAA regulations. |

*Note.* HIPAA=Health Insurance Portability and Accountability Act of 1996.

## Basic Demographic Information

Your patients' plastic insurance cards, which they should bring to their first meeting with you, contain most essential billing information. They should also call the mental health information number on their card and ask the questions listed below, the three most important of which are the following:

• If you have a provider network, is this clinician in the network?
• Do I need an authorization for outpatient treatment?
• To what address should mental health claims be mailed [if you submit paper claims]?

If you employ a billing service, its employees can collect this information if you give them a copy of both sides of the card. On the other hand, patients make better decisions about their treatment if they understand their insurance benefit. You may fax them a complete list of questions to ask their insurer (Appendix 6–C).

Collect the following information first:

• Patient's insurance ID number (a mistaken digit will probably cause a claims rejection)

- Patient's name (mistakes in this and most other data elements will not usually trigger a claims rejection, so long as the appropriate box on a claims form is not left blank)
- Patient's address
- Patient's date of birth
- Patient's sex
- Patient's telephone number
- Insurance subscriber's name, address, and date of birth

## Benefit Information

The insurance card often lists a co-pay amount, which the patient must pay for each session, next to the letters MH or OV. It also lists an 800 number for calling the insurer about general or mental health questions, and it is this 800 number that you should urge your patient to call for the following, additional information:

- Whether their insurer lists you in its provider network and how this affects payment for your services
- Whether the patient must pay an out-of-pocket deductible at the start of each year before their insurance makes its first payment
- How much co-pay their insurance requires them to pay for each treatment session
- Whether their insurer requires them or you to obtain prior authorization before treatment and, if so,
- How many sessions it will authorize initially and what must you do to obtain authorization for additional sessions
- To what address you should send your claims (knowing that the claims address on the insurance card is often for medical, and not mental health, claims)
- Whether their insurer has a policy denying payment if claims or an authorization arrive too late to meet a "timely filing limit"
- Whether, if patients receive mental health treatment from another clinician in addition to yourself, their insurer deducts the other clinician's services from the number it has authorized for treatment with you and vice versa
- Whether, if patients have a "parity" diagnosis of mental illness, the insurer's mental health benefit will pay for or authorize more sessions in a year or reimburse them at a higher rate than it would for nonparity diagnoses
- Whether certain diagnoses, such as a learning problem or mental retardation, are excluded from coverage

- Whether the insurer may refuse to authorize outpatient treatment if, after reviewing the clinical information you provide, it decides that treatment is not "medically necessary"

Here is what you need to know about each of these questions.

## The Significance of Provider Networks

Patients should ask: Is this clinician in-network? How does that affect what I pay? Here are four reasons they need to have this information before your first meeting:

1. Many patients will not wish to engage your services unless their insurer lists you as an "in-network provider" because their insurer will otherwise pay less or nothing, leaving the patient to pay more or all of your fee.
2. If an insurer does not have a provider network or if your patient wishes to see you regardless of the added cost, you may simplify your administrative tasks by billing your usual fee to the patient and asking him or her to pay you directly and manage all communications with the insurer.
3. Many kinds of "indemnity insurance" do not use networks and permit you to bill for the balance between your usual fee and the insurance payment. Planned provider organization (PPO) insurance pays for services by out-of-network clinicians, but patients must usually pay a higher co-pay than they would otherwise.
4. If patients tell you that they cannot find an in-network clinician, advise them that their managed insurer must either help them find one or provide the same support for an out-of-network referral.

## Deductible

A deductible is an amount that some insurance policies exclude from coverage at the beginning of each year, obliging patients to pay 100% of your allowable fees until they have paid that amount, at which point their insurance begins to pay. Patients should ask: What's my annual deductible, and has any of it been used yet this year by either medical or mental health services?

## Co-Pays

A co-pay is an out-of-pocket fee that patients must pay for each session once the cost of your services exceeds the annual deductible. The insurer sets the co-pay as either a fixed amount or a percentage of your fee. You may be mandated by your contract with the insurer to collect the co-pay, regardless of whether you believe the patient can afford it. Patients should ask: What is my co-pay?

## Prior and Concurrent Authorizations

As noted earlier, patients should determine whether their insurer requires that your services be "authorized" and whether an authorization is necessary for their first visit. They can do this without disclosing any clinical information by calling the 800 number on the back of their insurance card. The authorization will cover 4 to 12 treatment sessions in addition to 1 or 2 evaluation sessions (code 90801). An increasing number of insurers do not require authorization for initial evaluations or services performed uniquely by psychiatrists, such as "medication visits" (code 90862). Patients should also ask: How many sessions will this authorization cover? Is it needed for medication visits? Is there an expiration date?

## Mental Health Claims Address

Patients should confirm the address to which paper mental health claims should be sent, if you send them, because the claims address on the insurance card does not necessarily apply to mental health claims. In addition, many large national insurers have a different claims address for each of their insurance products. Patients should ask: To what address does my mental health claim need to be mailed?

## Timely Filing Deadlines

For reasons described previously, patients should ask: Is there a timely filing limit on authorizations or claims?

## Benefit Depletion by Another Clinician

If two clinicians provide concurrent treatment and the insurer puts an annual limit on the number of services or limits both treatments with one authorization, then services provided by one clinician may reduce the amount of coverage available for services provided by the other, and both clinicians may underestimate the number of sessions remaining available for coverage. You need to know whether the insurer lumps both treatments under the same authorization or annual benefit limit and, if so, whether certain psychiatric codes or substance abuse codes are exempt. Patients should ask: Will increasing my sessions with one of my clinicians reduce the number of sessions available for my other clinician, either the sessions currently authorized or the maximum number available for the coming year? If that is the case: Would this be true if one of my clinicians is a psychiatrist who uses a psychiatric billing code, specifically 90862, 90805, or 90807? Will it be true if one of my clinicians is a substance abuse counselor?

## Eligibility by Diagnosis

Most insurance benefits provide greater coverage for certain conditions, such as the following:

- Biologically based mental illnesses such as schizophrenia, affective illness, OCD, and anxiety disorder
- Dangerous behaviors such as suicide attempts or assaultiveness
- Childhood behaviors interfering with performance at school or safety at home

State laws often mandate insurers to provide more resources for certain mental illnesses than for other conditions, but these laws do not necessarily apply to all policies, particularly when large businesses self-insure. Your patient needs to determine whether parity regulations, making the same resources available for mental as for medical illness, apply to his or her benefit. You should know whether your state mandates a parity benefit and, if so, which diagnoses are covered. Most statutory lists of "biologically based mental illnesses" include schizophrenia and affective disorders, and some include eating disorders, anxiety disorders, and childhood behavioral disorders. Patients should ask: Are there certain diagnoses that entitle me to more services? What are they? Do they reduce the authorization process for ongoing treatment?

Patients should also know that most mental health insurance benefits specifically exclude coverage for conditions that require primarily educational or supportive care, such as mental retardation, autism, learning problems, conduct disorders, dementia, and other chronic medical and neurologic problems. Of course, the existence of one of these conditions does not preclude the patient's having a concurrent, acute psychiatric problem that is eligible for coverage.

## Medical Necessity

Managed insurance benefits, as noted earlier, may deny payment for any service that is not "medically necessary." Your patient should ask: Is coverage limited to medically necessary services?

## #3: Choose Your Billing Code

In contrast to "E and M" (evaluation and management) billing codes that provide nonpsychiatric physicians with a large number of rates and codes for outpatient medical services, the CPT (current procedural terminology) codes for outpatient mental health services are few and do not offer higher rates for complex services. For nonprescribing mental health clinicians, there are basically six codes: 90801 for a 1-hour diagnostic interview; 90804 for psychotherapy, 20–30 minutes; 90806 for psychotherapy, 45–50 minutes; 90846 or 90847 for family therapy; and 90853 for group psychotherapy. Psychiatrists can use three additional codes, as noted above under "Benefit Depletion by Another Clinician": 90862 for an approximately 15-minute "medication management visit"; 90805 for 20–30 minutes of psychotherapy with medication management; and 90807 for 45–50 minutes of psychotherapy with medication management. Recently, several insurers have begun to offer additional codes, after special authorization, for crisis services that last longer than 60 minutes. Determine what you feel is the fair code for the services you provide and inform your patient of the likely impact on his or her benefit. Table 6–2 compares medical and nonmedical codes.

You have a choice when a service might fall into more than one category. Practically speaking, this occurs for prescribing clinicians only, who will prefer to use the higher-paying 90805 or 90807 codes over the 90862. If, however, the patient who receives concurrent psychotherapy from another provider has an insurance benefit that lumps 90805 and 90807 codes together with the 90804 and 90806 codes used by the nonprescribing clinician, then the prescribing clinician's choice to use the higher-paying codes may accelerate depletion of the patient's psychotherapy benefit. Obviously, the prescribing clinician may feel that the higher fee is fair and yet may accept a lower fee to protect the patient's resources. For example, you might explain to the patient:

> "The code I will use to bill your insurer for my psychiatric services is for medication and psychotherapy, rather than for medication alone, because our sessions tend to last longer than 15 minutes and involve complex issues. Unfortunately, this may impose a greater paperwork burden on your therapist, who will need to obtain authorizations more frequently. If your benefit limits psychotherapy treatment sessions to a certain maximum a year, my sessions will also count against that number."

If sessions occur on an emergency basis and/or last longer than an hour, seek authorization from the insurer for a special, more highly reimbursed code or, if such a code is not offered, for an additional 90801, the code for a diagnostic interview. For Medicare patients, psychiatrists may be able to use "E and M codes" for such visits.

## #4: Collect Payment When Services Are Delivered

Know how much your patients should pay for each session and collect payment when services are delivered. Requiring patients to pay deductibles

TABLE 6–2.    Mental health service codes, highlighting options for prescribing clinicians

| Code | Advantages | Disadvantages |
|---|---|---|
| **For prescribing clinicians** | | |
| **90862** "medication management," 15 minutes or less | • Many insurers do not require authorization for this code.<br>• It usually does not reduce the number of sessions available for psychotherapy. | • Usually pays less than 90804 or 90805, and thus underpays when treatment requires more than 15 minutes. |
| **90805** medication plus psychotherapy, 20–30 minutes | • Pays more than 90862. | • Often requires authorization.<br>• May reduce number of sessions available for psychotherapy. |
| **90807** medication plus psychotherapy, 40–50 minutes | | • Often requires authorization.<br>• May reduce number of sessions available for psychotherapy |
| **For all clinicians** | | |
| **90801** diagnostic interview, 50 minutes | | • Usually requires authorization, but authorization is automatic. |
| **90804** psychotherapy, 25 minutes | | • May require authorization.<br>• Reduces number of sessions as much as if it were an hour-long session. |
| **90806** psychotherapy, 45–50 minutes | | • Requires authorization.<br>• Reduces number of sessions available for psychotherapy. |
| **90846** family psychotherapy | | • Requires authorization.<br>• Reduces number of sessions available for psychotherapy. |
| **90853** group psychotherapy | | • Requires authorization.<br>• Reduces number of sessions available for psychotherapy. |

and co-pays on a pay-as-you-go basis helps them anticipate expenses, avoid unexpected charges, and become more active in negotiating the potential cost of long-term treatment. Collecting during sessions reduces your overhead and improves the collection rate. Certain insurers, such as Medicare, may legally oblige you to make these collections. For instance, you might say to your patient, during the first session, "I'd appreciate your paying for the uncovered portion of your fees at the time of our session, by check or in cash" (or by credit card, if you have the capacity).

## #5: Notify Patients of Noncovered Items You Expect Them to Pay For

Notify patients, in advance, if you expect them to pay for any of the following:

- Missed appointments
- Call-in or mail-in prescriptions
- Written reports
- Copies of records
- Telephone calls

These are time-consuming events that are not covered by insurance. Appendix 6–D is a sample patient notification form that covers items listed above.

## #6: Screen for Parity Eligibility and for Noncovered Conditions

Screen patients for diagnoses that entitle them to "parity" benefits and document your findings. Also screen them for conditions that may not be covered. Diagnoses that may be eligible for additional benefits, or exempt from benefits, are described above under "Eligibility by Diagnosis."

## #7: Determine What Is Medically Necessary

To arrive at your own definition of medically necessary treatment, determine the following:

- The severity of the patient's condition, in terms of symptoms, behaviors, or disability
- The least costly intervention that will provide a result that meets your standards of safety and effectiveness

- The presence or absence of resources, other than insurance, that can be expected to provide care, such as family support, veterans' benefits, and educational entitlements.

Whenever possible, find evidence that less-than-recommended treatment will lead to a substandard result.

## #8: Discuss Medical Necessity With the Patient

Explain to your patient how you came to think that a particular treatment was medically necessary, work toward an agreement on this issue, and promise to update your agreement regularly. As noted under Principle #3 above, patients must be partners in determining how much treatment is medically necessary. Explore what they know about their insurance benefit and the meaning of "medical necessity" and fill in gaps in their knowledge. Describe your recommended treatment plan, explain why it is medically necessary, and invite comment and disagreement. Your patients need to know that their insurance benefits have limits and that you are trying to work within those limits to get them what they need and are entitled to, while avoiding costs that might fall on them to pay. For example, you might explain as follows:

> "Your insurance is unlikely to cover long-term treatment for your son's ag-gressive behavior because it is primarily due to mental retardation, which is not a covered condition. We can expect coverage for weekly outpatient treatment for at least a limited period of time whenever we need to change medication or respond to a crisis, or if it appears that a slow-down in treat-ment causes relapse."

You will often need to explain the conditions that make a long-term treatment medically necessary. For example:

> "Your insurance will probably not cover outpatient treatment for very long unless it appears to be protecting you from relapsing into a dangerous state, and it will not cover frequent sessions unless you appear to relapse every time the frequency of your sessions is reduced."

You will often need to explain how diagnosis affects medical necessity:

> "Your insurance benefit does not give a high priority to the treatment of marital conflict, but depression carries more weight, particularly when, as in your case, there is a history of a suicide attempt and hospital admission. Given that you now have symptoms of depression and that your marital conflict is likely to trigger relapse, I believe your insurance company will probably cover regular sessions once it knows your diagnosis, at least until your symptoms improve."

You may sometimes need to explain the difference between more and less costly options. For instance:

> "Unless you feel you'll be unsafe, we don't need to meet next week. Your managed insurance benefit is a 'no frills' policy that covers treatment that is necessary to protect your safety and restore you to your usual health, but nothing more. I believe we can put off meeting for a couple weeks without slowing down your progress, but you should definitely call me if you feel unsafe."

## #9: Track Claims and Authorizations to Avoid Timely-Filing Limits

If you do not use a billing service, use software that identifies charges that have gone unpaid for more than 60 days and authorizations that need to be renewed. If one uses a billing service, this tracking of lost payments and authorizations comprises a large part of the service's value. As a last resort, if you do your own billing, be prepared to offer proof of your having submitted a claim on time, such as a log of a monthly claims run, in order to obtain payment.

## #10: Anticipate the December 31 Deadline for Authorization Renewals

If many of your patients have the same insurer and their authorizations expire on December 31, ask the insurer whether it offers a short cut for reauthorizing ongoing treatment for a large number of patients. Some insurers will waive their reauthorization requirement for the first few sessions at the beginning of every year. Others streamline the process by allowing clinicians to send in a list of patients with their insurance numbers, diagnoses, and the kinds of sessions needed, rather than requiring them to complete an "Outpatient Treatment Report" (OTR) on each continuing case.

## #11: Document Evidence for Insurance Eligibility and Medical Necessity

If you treat many patients covered by one insurer, the insurer may wish to audit your charts and may rescind payment if the treatment does not seem medically necessary. This happens frequently with Medicaid and less often with private insurers. Your patients are entitled to ask you to redact (black out) information related to therapy. The insurer is entitled to view a copy of all other information documenting your services.

Be aware that the information insurers require is limited to the two issues described above: eligibility by diagnosis and medical necessity. Documenting medical necessity is best done by addressing evidence of risk of harm, threats to basic functioning, and responsiveness (or not) to prior treatment, and need not include any other personal details or information about the interpersonal process of treatment. For instance, to document the evidence of a mental illness or dangerous behavioral problem, it is less useful to write, "The patient is depressed about family and marital issues and in conflict about his passivity or aggression." It is more useful to write: "The patient has a 3-month history of increasing depression with tearfulness, diminished concentration, and job jeopardy due to poor performance." Or, to document the "restorative potential" of treating someone who has not been cured by prior treatment, it is less useful to write, "The patient needs intensive treatment because he has severe, long-standing symptoms." It is more useful to write, "He is likely to need weekly treatment during acute episodes because symptoms worsen rapidly and he develops suicide plans if he is seen less frequently." Clinicians who are unfamiliar with the concept of documenting medical necessity may find it helpful to read *Concise Guide to Managing Behavioral Health Care Within a Managed Care Environment* (Bennett 2002).

## ▌ CONCLUSION

Knowing how to bill insurers, particularly for managed benefits, will help you recover the payment you deserve, use your time for clinical rather than administrative tasks, and reduce overhead expenses. It will also help your patients make effective use of their benefits. In the long run, you need to understand the current system's wastefulness, unfairness, and inefficiency if you are to conceptualize improvements and advocate for reform.

## ▌ REFERENCE

Bennett MI: Concise Guide to Managing Behavioral Health Care Within a Managed Care Environment. Washington, DC, American Psychiatric Publishing, 2002

## APPENDIX 6–A

# HCFA 1500 Form, Common Data Requirements

PLEASE DO NOT STAPLE IN THIS AREA

**HEALTH INSURANCE CLAIM FORM**

| | |
|---|---|
| 1a. INSURED'S I.D. NUMBER | XXB41532346 |
| 2. PATIENT'S NAME | DOE JOHN W |
| 3. PATIENT'S BIRTH DATE | 10 10 90  SEX F X |
| 4. INSURED'S NAME | DOE JOHN W |
| 5. PATIENT'S ADDRESS | 324 MAPLE STREET |
| 6. PATIENT RELATIONSHIP TO INSURED | Spouse X |
| 7. INSURED'S ADDRESS | 324 MAPLE STREET |
| CITY | MIDDLEVILLE  STATE MA |
| 9. PATIENT STATUS | Other X |
| CITY | MIDDLEVILLE  STATE MA |
| ZIP CODE 02556 | TELEPHONE ( 555 ) 325 1460 |
| ZIP CODE 02556 | TELEPHONE ( 555 ) 325 1460 |
| 9. OTHER INSURED'S NAME | NONE |
| a. INSURED'S DATE OF BIRTH | 10 10 90  SEX F X |
| d. INSURANCE PLAN NAME OR PROGRAM NAME | BLUE SHIELD OF MASSACHUSETTS |
| 12. PATIENT'S OR AUTHORIZED PERSON'S SIGNATURE | SIGNATURE ON FILE  DATE 05 17 04 |
| 13. INSURED'S OR AUTHORIZED PERSON'S SIGNATURE | SIGNATURE ON FILE |
| 21. DIAGNOSIS OR NATURE OF ILLNESS OR INJURY | 1. 296.30 |
| 23. PRIOR AUTHORIZATION NUMBER | ABCD |

| 24. DATE(S) OF SERVICE From | To | Place of Service | Type of Service | PROCEDURES, SERVICES, OR SUPPLIES CPT/HCPCS | MODIFIER | DIAGNOSIS CODE | $ CHARGES | DAYS OR UNITS | | | | | RESERVED FOR LOCAL USE |
|---|---|---|---|---|---|---|---|---|---|---|---|---|---|
| 05 01 04 | | 3 | 9 | 90801 | | 296.30 | 175.00 | 1 | | | | | BE M0214 |
| 05 10 04 | | 3 | 1 | 90807 | | 296.30 | 175.00 | 1 | | | | | BE M0214 |
| 05 17 04 | | 3 | 1 | 90862 | | 296.30 | 85.00 | 1 | | | | | BE M0214 |

| 25. FEDERAL TAX I.D. NUMBER | 26. PATIENT'S ACCOUNT NO. | 27. ACCEPT ASSIGNMENT | 28. TOTAL CHARGE | 29. AMOUNT PAID | 30. BALANCE DUE |
|---|---|---|---|---|---|
| 415342514  X | 1853 | X YES | $ 435 00 | $ | $ |

31. SIGNATURE OF PHYSICIAN OR SUPPLIER
05 17 04

32. NAME AND ADDRESS OF FACILITY WHERE SERVICES WERE RENDERED

33. (617) 738-9204
FRED CLINICIAN
45 CEDAR ROAD
CHESTNUT HILL MA 02467-2209
BE M0214

PLEASE PRINT OR TYPE

APPROVED OMB-0938-0008 FORM CMS-1500 (12-90), FORM RRB-1500,
APPROVED OMB-1215-0055 FORM OWCP-1500, APPROVED OMB-0720-0001 (CHAMPUS)

## APPENDIX 6–B

# HCFA 1500 Form, Medicare Data Requirements

PLEASE DO NOT STAPLE IN THIS AREA

**HEALTH INSURANCE CLAIM FORM**

| | | | | | |
|---|---|---|---|---|---|
| 1a. INSURED'S I.D. NUMBER | | | | | XXB41532346 |

2. PATIENT'S NAME: DOE JOHN W

3. PATIENT'S BIRTH DATE: 10 10 90  SEX M [X] F

4. INSURED'S NAME: DOE JOHN W

5. PATIENT'S ADDRESS: 324 MAPLE STREET

6. PATIENT RELATIONSHIP TO INSURED: Self [X]

7. INSURED'S ADDRESS: 324 MAPLE STREET

CITY: MIDDLEVILLE  STATE: MA

8. PATIENT STATUS: Other [X]

CITY: MIDDLEVILLE  STATE: MA

ZIP CODE: 02556  TELEPHONE: (555) 325 1460

ZIP CODE: 02556  TELEPHONE: (555) 325 1460

9. OTHER INSURED'S NAME: NONE

10. IS PATIENT'S CONDITION RELATED TO:

11. INSURED'S POLICY GROUP OR FECA NUMBER

a. OTHER INSURED'S POLICY OR GROUP NUMBER

a. EMPLOYMENT? (CURRENT OR PREVIOUS) YES [ ] NO [X]

a. INSURED'S DATE OF BIRTH: 10 10 90  SEX M [ ] F [X]

b. OTHER INSURED'S DATE OF BIRTH

b. AUTO ACCIDENT? YES [ ] NO [X]  PLACE (State)

b. EMPLOYER'S NAME OR SCHOOL NAME

c. EMPLOYER'S NAME OR SCHOOL NAME

c. OTHER ACCIDENT? YES [ ] NO [X]

c. INSURANCE PLAN NAME OR PROGRAM NAME: BLUE SHIELD OF MASSACHUSETTS

d. INSURANCE PLAN NAME OR PROGRAM NAME

10d. RESERVED FOR LOCAL USE

d. IS THERE ANOTHER HEALTH BENEFIT PLAN? YES [X] NO [ ]

12. PATIENT'S OR AUTHORIZED PERSON'S SIGNATURE: SIGNATURE ON FILE  DATE 05 17 04

13. INSURED'S OR AUTHORIZED PERSON'S SIGNATURE: SIGNATURE ON FILE

21. DIAGNOSIS OR NATURE OF ILLNESS OR INJURY: 1. 296.30

23. PRIOR AUTHORIZATION NUMBER: ABCD

| 24. A. DATE(S) OF SERVICE From / To | B. Place of Service | C. Type of Service | D. PROCEDURES, SERVICES, OR SUPPLIES CPT/HCPCS / MODIFIER | E. DIAGNOSIS CODE | F. $ CHARGES | G. DAYS OR UNITS | H. EPSDT Family Plan | I. EMG | J. COB | K. RESERVED FOR LOCAL USE |
|---|---|---|---|---|---|---|---|---|---|---|
| 05 01 04 | 3 | 9 | 90801 | 296.30 | 175.00 | 1 | | | | BE M0214 |
| 05 10 04 | 3 | 1 | 90807 | 296.30 | 175.00 | 1 | | | | BE M0214 |
| 05 17 04 | 3 | 1 | 90862 | 296.30 | 85.00 | 1 | | | | BE M0214 |

25. FEDERAL TAX I.D. NUMBER: 415342514 [X]

26. PATIENT'S ACCOUNT NO.: 1853

27. ACCEPT ASSIGNMENT? YES [X] NO [ ]

28. TOTAL CHARGE: $ 435 00

31. SIGNATURE OF PHYSICIAN OR SUPPLIER: MICHAEL BENNETT, M.D.  05 17 04

32. NAME AND ADDRESS OF FACILITY WHERE SERVICES WERE RENDERED: FRED CLINICIAN  214 TREATMENT STREET  MEADOWRIDGE MA 13142

33. PHYSICIAN'S, SUPPLIER'S BILLING NAME, ADDRESS, ZIP CODE: (617) 738-9204  FRED CLINICIAN  45 CEDAR ROAD  CHESTNUT HILL MA 02467-2209  BE M0214

PLEASE PRINT OR TYPE

APPENDIX 6–C

# Sample Information Sheet: Understanding Your Insurance Benefit

We need to understand how much your insurance is likely to pay for treatment if we are to predict how much it may cost you. Your insurance card, which you should bring to our first session, will tell us your identification number, but prior to our first meeting you should contact your insurer directly, using the 800 number on your card, to find out the following:

- Whether your insurer includes me in its clinician network and, if not, how much this will reduce your coverage
- Whether you must pay an out-of-pocket "deductible" at the start of each year before your insurance makes its first payment
- How much "co-pay" your insurance expects you to pay for each treatment session
- Whether your insurer requires you or me to contact them and obtain "prior authorization" prior to treatment and, if so,
- How many sessions it will authorize initially and what it will require you or me to do to obtain authorization for additional sessions
- To what address I should send your claims (knowing that the claims address on your insurance card is often for medical, and not mental health, claims)
- Whether their insurer imposes a "timely filing limit" that denies payment if we request authorization after, rather than before, performing services or delay in filing a claim and, if so, how long these limits are
- Whether, if you receive mental health treatment from another clinician in addition to myself, your insurer will deduct the other clinician's services from the number it has authorized for treatment with me or vice versa

Ask your insurer whether your insurance benefit is "managed." (It certainly is if your insurer requires authorization.) If it is, you will need to ask me how my clinical findings will affect your coverage. This is best done after I have completed an initial evaluation. Meanwhile, ask your insurer:

- Whether, if you have a "parity" diagnosis of mental illness, the insurer will pay for more sessions or authorize more sessions at a time than it would otherwise
- Whether certain diagnoses, such as a learning problem or mental retardation, are excluded from coverage

- Whether the insurer may refuse to authorize outpatient treatment if, after reviewing the clinical information you provide, it decides that treatment is not "medically necessary"

If you have "managed" insurance, ask me about "medical necessity." The best way to obtain coverage for "medically necessary" treatment is to work out our own plan for what we consider "medically necessary" treatment before your insurer attempts to impose its own definition. To be medically necessary, a treatment must be the least costly way of either improving your condition or preventing it from worsening. Thus, we can only consider treatments that have proven themselves scientifically and we cannot use a more costly treatment if a less costly one is likely to do the job. We can always choose to pursue treatments that are not classified as "medically necessary," but if we do so, we cannot expect your insurance to cover it. After I have completed an evaluation, we will prepare a plan for medically necessary treatment and also discuss alternatives.

## APPENDIX 6–D

# Sample Notice to Patients Regarding Cost of Ancillary Services

### ▮ MISSED APPOINTMENTS

Missed appointments are charged to patients at my usual, private, nondiscounted fee (please ask) unless they are unavoidable or I receive 24 hours notice. Please note: my fee is not equivalent to an insurance co-payment.

### ▮ CALL-IN PRESCRIPTIONS

Call-in prescriptions are charged to patients at $10 per regular prescription, $20 per controlled-substance prescription, unless we have discussed them in advance and consider them unavoidable.

### ▮ REPORTS

The time required to compose disability and other reports is charged to patients at my regular, nondiscounted fee (please ask) unless they are paid for by the party requesting the report or can be done during a clinical session. I decline to do reports for legal purposes, such as establishing grounds for a personal injury claim.

### ▮ COPIES

There is no charge to patients for a copy of their record for their own use; copies for other purposes are charged to patients at my regular, nondiscounted fee (please ask) unless the party requesting the report pays for them.

### ▮ SHARING YOUR RECORD WITH YOUR PRIMARY CARE PHYSICIAN

Please sign a consent form allowing me to share your record with your primary care physician (assuming that you wish me to) and give me your primary care physician's fax number.

### ▮ TELEPHONE CALLS

Page me only in emergencies. There is no charge for necessary calls—that is, calls about side effects, the presence of severe symptoms, lost medication, or the need for a change in treatment, although I may need to see you face to face before I can respond. The time required for other calls is charged to patients at my regular, nondiscounted fee (please ask).

REFERENCE

Bennett MI: *A Concise Guide to Managing Behavioral Health Care Within a Managed Care Environment*. Washington, DC, American Psychiatric Publishing, 2002

# 7

# COMPUTER RESOURCES FOR THE PRIVATE PRACTICE

*John Luo, M.D.*

The private practice setting offers many opportunities for computer-based applications as well as some novel approaches. There are many technological innovations that can simplify scheduling, enable you to document encounters while away from the office, or even check patient records securely on your handheld computer. Whether the practice consists of one practitioner or a group, a variety of innovative technology solutions exist that can facilitate many activities in private practice.

New technologies should not be used just for new technologies' sake. The ideas described in this chapter serve to improve the quality of patient care by minimizing the administrative overhead or enhancing clinical services. Although some ideas may save only a few minutes in the day, others may avoid patient care emergencies by extending the reach of the therapeutic relationship. With the extent to which advances in information technology have permeated society, it is hard to imagine medical practice without a computer.

There are varying levels of complexity for the computing solutions described in this chapter. They range from actions simple enough for even the novice computer user to those that are challenging even for the technologically savvy. None of these ideas requires a Ph.D. in computer science to implement, but the range of requisite computing knowledge is quite varied. Limits on time and willingness to learn are more likely to be obstacles, and they may lead you to consider outsourcing the computer services by hiring a consultant.

A key frame of reference in considering the computing solutions presented in this chapter is to ask the question "How does this fit within how I practice?" If you stay in one office and never need access to your records while off site, then a pager may be the only technology you will need. In another scenario, if you visit a different clinic for several days a week, then a notebook computer with linkages to the main data repository may be sufficient. There is nothing more frustrating than to invest time and money in a technology solution only to have it fail because considerations of workplace culture and habits have been omitted.

The topics in this chapter are organized in an "outside the office to inside the office" structure. First, the various issues and potential implications for a Web site will be discussed, ranging from advertising to scheduling and patient screening. Next, patient waiting area ideas such as wireless Internet access, information kiosks, and solutions for gathering patients' demographic information will be explored. Turning to factors inside the office, the various technologies for documentation, billing, and medical reference, as well as their security implications, will be reviewed. In a return to connection to the outside, novel technologies such as Web logs, telemedicine, and e-mail will highlight ways to enhance connectivity. Given the rapidly shifting nature of computer-based services, most of these ideas will be discussed in general to avoid references to outdated information; however, representative hardware or software companies will be mentioned as a resource starting point. Commonly used terms appear in **boldface** and are defined in the glossary at the end of the chapter.

## ▌ WEB SITE

Traditionally, most private practices are listed in the telephone book and referrals take place from other physicians or by way of lists sent to patients. In today's information technology age, the rich interconnectivity and interactivity of the Internet serves the physician, insurance company, and patient well. Depending on your level of computer expertise, the increasingly nationwide availability of fast Internet access via a **DSL** or **cable modem** can provide the infrastructure for more than just a home page.

Creating a Web site is easy nowadays, and knowledge of **HTML** is not even necessary. Programs such as Microsoft's FrontPage or Hotdog PageWiz help you create a Web page by taking care of the HTML code for you. Many Internet service providers offer Web site creation via templates, which are easy to use. If you wish to learn how to create an HTML page, go to a Web site such as PageResource.com (http://www.pageresource.com/html/index.html) or How-to-Build-Websites.com (http://www.how-to-build-websites.com) and read the basic tutorial. Although fancy graphics and navigational methods are usually a plus, it is the content that really drives people to a Web site. Dr. Robert Hsiung's psychopharmacology Web site (http://www.dr-bob.org) is an example of a site with an easily remembered domain name and a good balance of graphics and text.

Once you have created your Web site, the next step is to find a "host." This company may be your Internet service provider (**ISP**), which provides you with space on their **server** to run your Web site, or it may be a separate **Web hosting** company such as myhosting.com. Typical costs for Internet access depend on speed and server space but average around $50 a month. If you wish to have your own **domain name**, such as http://www.psymd.com, you will have to register your name with a domain name service such as Internic, which may cost anywhere between $20 and $40 per year. This service is necessary because your server has an **internet protocol** (**IP**) address— a number, for example 123.123.0.23, which is more difficult to remember than a name. Choosing an easy-to-recall domain name is important because it helps solidify your clinical identity and it is easier for people to remember.

If you have a **static IP address** (a number that is assigned to you and therefore doesn't change each time you connect to the Internet) from your ISP, you could even host your own site on your computer at the office, using a Web server program such as Apache (http://www.apache.org). However, this process is recommended only to practitioners with more advanced computer skills, a sufficiently powerful computer to handle the demand for requests, and the willingness to deal with other issues such as backup, power outages, and capacity. Most physicians will likely outsource their Web site to a Web hosting consulting firm such as 1EZConsulting to deal with these issues as well as **DNS registration** and site design. A great way to find local firms is to use a search engine such as Google and enter [*city*] and *website consulting* as search terms.

Another way to avoid headaches is to use a service such as Medem (http://www.medem.com) to handle all of these issues. Medem is a company created by a consortium of medical societies to address the growing need of physicians to have a Web presence. If you are a member of the American Psychiatric Association, a Web site created via Medem is a member benefit. Using a Web browser to enter information into forms, you can quickly create a Web site via the templates provided by Medem. The **uniform resource locator** (**URL**) is quite easy to remember because it uses your name (example: http://www.uclapsychiatry.yourmd.com/Luo). The limitations of this service are that the site will be of a basic design and you will have limited control over the advertisements that appear as well as the patient resource documents listed. However, the infrastructure does provide a secure channel of electronic communication with your patients, which may be an important service. If you do not belong to a medical specialty society, the services at Medem currently cost $95 per year.

Many people have their own Web sites hosted at free services such as http://www.tripod.lycos.com or http://geocities.yahoo.com. Using these companies comes with a price, in that they will provide advertising on your Web site that is not within your control. These ads can have almost any content and will be located wherever on your site the free hosting company decides. In addition, the URL provided may also be rather long and obscure. It is very unprofessional to have your practice site hosted on this free service; however, it may be appropriate for nonprofit informational sites provided as a community service.

## Increasing Hits

Visibility of a Web site on the Internet does not depend on word of mouth alone. A *hit* is defined as a visit to your Web site from another computer. As is true of ads, a popular Web site will have many hits. One way to increase hits is to have links to your site from various referral portals. As with traditional advertising, many portals will list you for a set charge, and some sites will do it for free. For example, The American Medical Association (AMA) Physician Finder (http://dbapps.ama-assn.org/aps/amahg.htm) helps the public to find physicians, either by name or specialty, within a geographic region. Their database has the names of both AMA members and nonmembers, but AMA members' names appear higher on the generated list.

There are numerous doctor referral sites for patients to visit, and these also can be a source of new patient referrals for the practice. In addition, if you register for insurance panels, the insurance companies' Web sites will also list your practice. Many of the sites are interrelated, which means that for some sites, you need list your information only once. An example is that The Little Blue Book (http://www.tlbb.com) owns MDHub (http://www.mdhub.com), which provides free messaging for your site as well as WebMD (http://www.webmd.com) owns The Little Blue Book and uses information from that database. Other national listing services for doctors include LocateADoc (http://www.locateadoc.com), Doctor Directory (http://www.doctordirectory.com), and Doctor Page (http://www.doctorpage.com).

At this time, there are very few psychiatry-specific listing services, and most that do exist are general mental health listings. PsychSites (http://www.psychsites.com) is the only listing service that has primarily psychiatrists, although they are expanding to include other mental health professionals and to serve other major metropolitan areas. Other general sites on which to consider posting your site include Therapist Finder (http://www.therapistfinder.net), MentalHealth (http://www.mentalhealth.net), and Find-A-Psychiatrist (http://www.find-a-psychiatrist.com). Some of these sites will list your practice for free, but others charge a yearly fee.

Another mechanism to direct people to your Web site is to make use of search engines. The most popular one, Google (http://www.google.com), has a sophisticated search algorithm that is based primarily on a "rank" determined by the number of sites that provide a link back to your site. More links to your site will translate to a higher rank. This high rank is desirable because Web sites listed on the first page of search results are the ones most often seen. Another method to improve rank listing by search engines is frequent use of a key word on the Web site; however, attempts to cheat will be counted against your site. Many of these search engines will allow you to submit your site for free, such as Google (http://www.http://www.google.com/addurl.html). In addition, it is possible to pay for higher placement in the search information sent to the user. You can choose the terms that you wish to be linked with on Google (https://adwords.google.com/select/) and thus have your site listed higher in a search. These techniques can be used to increase your Web site presence, but they are probably not necessary. It is more likely (and preferable) that you will get referrals from other physicians and from your existing patients than from random patients surfing the Internet.

## Online Functions

There are many advantages to using a Web site to provide services for your patients. For example, many physicians use a Web site to provide information such as descriptions of different illnesses, their treatment, and their prognosis. If your Web site is hosted by Medem, the company uses material provided by the American Psychiatric Association. It is a common practice to include links to Web sites that provide additional information of value to patients. However, links move people away from your Web site. It is better to use **Javascript** (get examples at javascript.internet.com) to open a new browser for these links.

In addition to providing information, a Web site can gather information from your patients. Prospective patients can fill out forms with insurance information or even screening questionnaires to help identify their issues (see http://www.depression-screening.org/screeningtest/screeningtest.htm for an example). Once treatment is established, patients can log in and fill out rating scales to provide a measure of their treatment progress (see http://www.psychcorpcenter.com). The setup of such a Web-based database system is best outsourced to a computer professional because of the complex data management needs and security concerns. One popular way to find a part-time or contract programmer is to use Craigslist (http://www.craigslist.org), an online bulletin board where jobs can be posted for free in many major cities (but not in San Francisco). Another way to find relatively inexpensive computer talent is to check with your local university to see if they have a student-run Web design consultation service. For more professional and experienced programmers, Web site consulting firms are recommended.

With the increasing Internet savvy of the general public, patients may be ready for online scheduling software. Timing Corporation (http://www.timingcorp.com), Appointment Quest (http://www.appointmentquest.com), and SCI Systems (http://www.scheduling.com) offer software to provide this service online, and some work even with a **kiosk**, which is a standalone computer system designed to be used by the average person with little computer experience (http://www.kiosks.org/faq.html). Such software provides for online or kiosk-based registration, payment of co-pay via credit card, and appointment scheduling. Various rules prevent or allow double-booking as well as longer appointments for specific patients. Patients are able to see only the available appointments slots and cannot access information regarding other patients. These sites indicate that the software is HIPAA compliant with adequate 128-bit security and privacy measures guarding access to information. (For discussion of HIPAA, see the "Security" section under "Office" later in this chapter, as well as Chapter 9 of this volume.)

# ▮ WAITING ROOM

## Information Resources

In most offices, while patients are waiting to be seen they read magazines available in the waiting room or literature regarding various disorders and treatment. This traditional approach is well accepted; however, the magazines may last only a few months, and literature may become outdated. A novel approach would be to use an information kiosk or tablet PC to deliver information or even to collect data. The kiosk (see http://www.affordablekiosks.com for examples) offers the advantage of a system that can be easily secured physically, whereas a tablet PC provides more portability but poses a significant security challenge.

Patient information may be delivered either through access to a CD-

ROM library hosted by the office server or through a PowerPoint presentation. If office space permits, a separate area for a desktop computer or kiosk offers patients a great information resource or a chance to catch up on their e-mail. Alternatively, you can lend out CD-ROMs or print out resources from your office computer.

These computer-based information resources are best suited to an office that has front office staff to monitor and help the patients. Although these ideas can be implemented in a solo practice, the technical and security challenges may be too great. For the solo practitioner, many of these information resources should be made available on your Web site.

## Internet Access

Many of the established screening tools are available only on the Internet. One method is to have a **LAN** (local area network) setup in the office with connections via wires to computers available in the waiting room. Access to the main office server must be limited, and this is best done by limiting the privileges of the guest user accounts. Microsoft Windows 2000 and Windows XP have easily-created setup routines for guests, which limit their access to programs, hard drives, and choices of software.

Another idea for access is to provide **Wi-Fi** or wireless LAN access to the server and or the Internet. Many businesses such as airports and Starbucks coffee shops provide this service, but it would be novel for the physician to provide access in the waiting room. Wireless Internet is one of the fastest-growing technology sectors. Although it is confusing to keep up with the various versions, such as 802.11b, 802.11a, 802.11g, and so on, the 802.11b standard is sufficient for most offices. The range of 802.11b is about 20 feet if there are obstructions such as walls or several hundred feet without any obstructions. Even though the 802.11b transmission speed is not extremely fast, it is sufficient for most purposes. The prices of the wireless access points and wireless network adapters range from $50 to $100 depending on their features.

One of the important issues for the practice using Wi-Fi is to maintain sufficient security. Although the **WEP** (wireless encryption protocol) has been demonstrated be insecure, enabling it will be sufficient to keep the majority of users out of your network. In addition, disabling file sharing and leaving networked computers turned off at night will also prevent unauthorized access to your files. If your **wireless access point** permits this feature, limit which **MAC** (media access control) addresses have access to the network. Most wireless access points have built-in **routers**, which allow an Internet connection to be shared among several computers by routing information requests from the ISP to the designated computers on your network. Most routers have built-in **firewall** programs that monitor traffic with logs and can prevent unauthorized access. Finally, turning off the **SSID** (service set identifier) of your access points will make the connection harder to discover. Security cannot be emphasized enough when using wireless Internet in the health care setting. MAC address restriction, WEP enabling, and SSID turnoff should be sufficient for preventing unauthorized access to your Internet connection, and if file sharing is disabled, easy access to your data is eliminated.

Although it is unlikely that many psychiatrists will offer patients access to a wireless office network, such a network is quite practical for your own use. The obvious reason is that it avoids the time and effort spent to deploy wires throughout the office—and added wiring is not permitted by some office landlords. In a solo practitioner's office, a network may not be necessary, but in a group practice or shared space among individual practitioners, an office network makes economic sense and provides for information sharing.

One of the compelling reasons to offer wireless Internet connections to your patients is that it may indeed increase timely arrival for appointments because the patients know they can check their e-mail at your office. If you do offer Web surfing to your patients, be sure to use a content filter such as Web Washer URL Filter (http://www.webwasher.com) or Cyber Patrol (http://www.cyberpatrol.com) so that someone else's browsing does not expose you to risks.

A very good reason to deploy a wireless Internet network is that it will enable the use a wireless camera in your waiting room. D-Link (http://www.dlink.com) and other companies offer a camera that will transmit video signals via radio waves. In contrast to the hard-wiring of a traditional camera system with connections to a television set, this camera permits viewing and recording on the office computer. The software limits access to the video to specified users only, and it allows control over pan and tilt to scan the room. These cameras range in cost from $150 up to $500 depending on their features. Although such use of technology sounds ominous, it makes sense to know who is in your waiting room when you are alone.

# ■ OFFICE

## Notebook Versus Desktop Computers

One of the more difficult decisions about office technology is whether to have a notebook computer or to use a desktop computer in the office. Many years ago, there was a performance sacrifice and a higher cost associated with a notebook computer, but with today's technological advances this gap is negligible to the business user. Which type of computer to choose is now a matter of preference.

An obvious advantage of a notebook computer is its portability. For psychiatrists who commute to several office locations or who speak on the road at many meetings, a notebook computer is an obvious choice. Docking stations and port replicators offer the ease of connecting to larger monitors, full-size keyboards, peripherals such as a mouse, and office networks with just one connection.

The size of the notebook computer depends on what your use pattern will be. There are three classes of notebooks: subnotebook, compact, and desktop replacement. The subnotebook computer typically is very light (about 3 pounds) but has a smaller screen size (less than 12 inches) and fewer integrated accessories. At the opposite extreme, the desktop-replacement notebook is heavier (usually more than 6 pounds) but has a larger screen (about 14 inches) and many integrated accessories such as a CD-ROM drive. The compact class falls in between these classes and offers a balance of size, weight, performance, and accessories.

Desktop computers offer significant advantages, such as more computing power and monitor size for less money. Although they lack portability, there are several ways to access information on desktop computers while away from the office. Software such as Symantec PC Anywhere (http://www.symantec.com) and services such as LogMeIn (http://www.logmein.com) or GoToMyPC (http://www.gotomypc.com) will allow you to control and access the desktop computer from any computer at home or in another location. These programs and services offer secure connections either via the Internet or modem.

Another way to transfer data between notebook and desktop computers is to use flash memory drives, also known as "jump" or "thumb" drives. These devices are not actually hard drives, but use flash RAM (random access memory) to store information. They plug into a USB (universal serial bus) port of the computer and are used just like a floppy disk. Many of them are small enough to be carried around on a key chain.

Flash drives are extremely portable and therefore pose a significant security risk. Any use of protected health information requires some security measures. Most manufacturers provide software to create a secured directory that is password protected. Some devices even have a built-in fingerprint reader for security. If your flash drive does not provide these security measures, use encryption software such as AxCrypt (http://axcrypt.sourceforge.net) for Windows computers and Crypt for Mac OS X (http://www.securemac.com/macosxcrypt.php).

## Personal Digital Assistants

For most physicians, a personal digital assistant (**PDA**) or handheld computer is an excellent way to have information at your fingertips when away from your computer. Although the small screen size of PDAs makes editing and reading text difficult, their numerous capabilities and their portability are outstanding. A PDA is an excellent choice for physicians on the go in the hospital or on the road at a meeting. After the therapy or medication management session, a PDA slips unobtrusively out of your pocket to schedule the next appointment.

In addition to basic personal information-management capabilities, what PDAs can do is limited only by your imagination. Reference texts such as DSM-IV-TR, drug information such as the *Physicians' Desk Reference* and ePocrates, and other materials are available for viewing. Medical calculators can determine the patient's body mass index and creatinine clearance. Portable keyboards and a PDA work well for document editing if it is needed on the go. Presentations can be delivered from your PDA, which is significantly lighter to carry than a notebook computer.

The two main operating systems of PDAs are Palm and Windows Mobile. Palm OS devices have better battery life and in general are easier to use. More medical software is available for Palm OS devices, but Windows Mobile devices typically have larger screens, can handle multimedia better, and are favored by large enterprises. In addition, there are combination PDA and mobile phone devices for both operating systems.

## Tablet PC

Tablet PCs are new devices that are finding increasing popularity. These computers offer the advantage of a "touch screen" built into the LCD panel, allowing use of a stylus to select/click items or even capture handwriting. Tablet PCs come in two types, the "slate" and the "convertible." The slate is designed to be primarily used as a touch screen device, and accessories such as a keyboard are attached separately. The convertible model looks like a normal notebook computer but has the additional ability to swivel the display 180 degrees and to be locked into place, hiding the keyboard.s

The advantage of using a tablet PC is that many electronic medical record software programs take advantage of the slate shape for data entry. The pen is a natural and easy way to select dropdown menus and click on buttons to enter demographic information or even generate progress notes with software such as ICANotes (http://www.icanotes.com). Check Web sites such as MedicalTabletPC (http://medicaltabletpc.com), Tablet-

PCBuzz (http://www.tabletpcbuzz.com), and TabletPCTalk (http://www.tabletpctalk.com) for more information.

## Placement

Where you locate the computer in the office depends on how you intend to use it in practice. If you intend to keep the computer available during sessions for patient education or to generate your notes during the visit, the physical location of the computer is quite important because typing on or reading from the computer diverts your attention from the patient.

When physicians type during the patient visit, some patients feel that they have been ignored or not taken seriously, whereas others may view the situation as a sign that what they have reported is significant and must be well documented. Other psychiatrists report that they do not use the computer during the session, but instead compose notes afterward. Use common sense and watch for nonverbal cues to understand how your computer use affects your relationships with your patients.

One advantage of using a notebook computer in a docking station is that during the patient session, the screen can be closed down. The notebook will then be in a hibernation state, and when needed, it can be quickly restarted where it left off. Similarly, a desktop computer screen can be blanked out by turning it off or setting the screen saver to blank. Screen savers nowadays are used more for entertainment value than for screen protection; they should be set to a blank screen during a session to avoid distractions.

## Scheduling

Various software programs are available to set up appointment schedules. Patients can be directed to use online scheduling software, or the physician can enter appointments directly into a calendar program such as Microsoft Outlook. An alternative is to use a PDA or handheld computer to setup an appointment in the calendar section; this is then synchronized with the office computer. The advantage of using this small device is that it is quickly turned on and its size does not significantly interfere with maintaining eye contact. One caveat is to ensure that this information is synchronized frequently to keep unwanted double-booking at a minimum. Programs such as "Therapist Helper" (http://www.helper.com) offer PDA-based interfaces with desktop software for this purpose. An alternative is that many billing system software packages offer an integrated calendar function that serves several purposes. Electronic medical record programs also offer this scheduling feature, and some will track insurance authorizations as well.

## Internet Service Providers

Obtaining health-related information has become one of the primary reasons that patients use the Internet. With today's more graphic-intensive Web sites and wealth of health-related information and misinformation, having Internet access is no longer a luxury but a business necessity for the physician.

Dial-up access to the Internet is adequate for many people, but the slow transmission speeds and frequent drops in connection with this type of access make a good argument for finding a **broadband** solution. This term is used to describe methods of receiving access at faster rates than dial-up modems, such as satellite, cable modem, and **DSL** (digital subscriber line). **ISDN** (integrated services digital network) also offered significantly faster speeds, but this technology has become obsolete.

Often the choice of broadband provider is limited to what is available in your area. In order to have cable or DSL, your office must be located sufficiently near the central office of your Internet provider. In more rural areas or areas without access, satellite or wireless Internet access are viable options. For those who can choose, DSL and cable access offer the best speeds for the cost per month, typically around $50. Most users typically download information more than they upload. If upload speed is important, you may need to pay more for a higher level of service.

The primary advantage of cable modem is that it offers high download and upload speeds, but these speeds are limited by the number of cable modem subscribers presently using the service. Cable modems users share the bandwidth available, so in areas of high cable modem density and peak usage, service can slow to a crawl. However, cable modem users typically enjoy both fast download and upload speeds.

DSL has the advantage of more dedicated access, but the speeds available are also in flux. The factors here are not the number of DSL users, but the quality of the telephone line and how distant your access is from the local telephone service provider. Keep in mind that many ISPs have different prices for the different download speeds, with a minimum speed guarantee. A dedicated phone line is not necessary for DSL, but any devices sharing the same phone line must be shielded with use of special phone line filters that are provided by your ISP.

Some ISPs offer support for the sharing of broadband access among multiple computers. The ISP provides router and switching equipment at low cost, with a monthly additional fee for helpdesk services. Although installation of the modem and router may appear rather daunting to the novice user, many companies such as 2Wire (http://www.2wire.com), D-Link (http://www.dlink.com), and Linksys (http://www.linksys.com) offer integrated solutions to make life easier. In fact, many of these setups are extremely simple even for the computer novice.

Networking does not require drilling holes to put in the Category 5 network cable throughout the office. You can avoid the difficulty by setting up a secure wireless network. Alternative network wiring solutions use the existing telephone jacks or power outlets in the office. The primary disadvantage of these latter solutions as opposed to wireless or Category 5 network cable is that transmission speeds are slower because of interference and poorer line quality.

Wireless networks are quite popular in today's businesses, but in addition to security, there are other factors to consider. Wireless access is dependent on radio waves to transmit the signal. Depending on the protocol used, this transmission spectrum is shared by other devices such as cordless telephones. The popular 2.4-GHz cordless telephone will certainly interfere with the 802.11b and 802.11g types of wireless Internet access, since they share the same frequency spectrum. In this situation, 802.11a, which is in the 5-GHz spectrum, will avoid such interference, but it is more expensive and has a limited range.

Radio signals are also affected by dense objects such as walls, which reduce signal strength. If there is a direct line of sight from the access point to the access client, you will have greater range. However, very thick and sturdy walls will limit both range and speed because they interfere with the signal. You should try to place the access point in a central location where it will reach the majority of computers. For the remaining computers, a device known as a **wireless repeater** can extend your signal range.

## Software

Certain software products are essential to the private practice. An office suite software package that has a word processor, spreadsheet program, database program, and presentation program is standard. Microsoft Office is almost a standard by default, but other suites such as Corel WordPerfect Office and Lotus SmartSuite work as well. One option to beat the high cost of these suites is to use Open Office (http://www.openoffice.org). This software package is compatible with Microsoft Office but does not have all of its features. It is free to use because of its open-source license.

In addition, there are times when a document must be preserved in its formatting. Adobe portable document format (**PDF**) is the standard used on the Internet. This file type is especially important when the recipient does not have the software program that created the file. The Adobe Acrobat software itself is useful for adding comments or editing PDFs, but otherwise, a free PDF converter such as PrimoPDF (http://www.primopdf.com)

or PDFCreator (http://www.sector7g.wurzel6.de/pdfcreator/index_en.htm) will work well. These products work by creating a virtual printer that then converts the print job into a PDF file.

## Document Entry

There are various methods to document patient care encounters using a computer. These methods offer significant advantages over the traditional handwritten note. When patients are treated either on an inpatient or an outpatient basis, much of the existing note can be carried forward to the next encounter in the electronic medium with a simple copy and paste. In situations where patients are seen only on a one-time basis this feature obviously does not apply, but there are a variety of methods to limit typing or hand-writing.

Today, speech recognition software has improved dramatically, attaining more than 95% accuracy for normal speech. Previously, the voice recognition hardware and software limitations required a slower pace and more pronounced speech in order to achieve decent accuracy. Software today such as IBM ViaVoice and Scansoft Dragon NaturallySpeaking (http://www.scansoft.com/viavoice) both have professional versions with specialized medical vocabularies to improve medical dictation recognition, albeit at higher costs. These speech recognition engines are quite sophisticated, and training can increase accuracy to 99%. Both ViaVoice and Dragon NaturallySpeaking offer the capability to dictate into separate voice recorders, but the Preferred Edition of Dragon NaturallySpeaking also permits dictation on Pocket PC PDAs, with transcription of these voice files on the desktop computer after transfer.

Traditional dictation services have also improved their offerings to include the capability of online transcription correction and multiple input methods such as dictation recorders, telephone, and PDAs. These services, such as Scribes Online (http://www.scribesonline.com), offer the ability to download corrected transcriptions for input into your medical record system. In addition to PDA-based entry, TalkNotes (http://www.provox.com/pv.asp?P=TNOver) has additional capability to enter information into customized forms. Macros are voice command shortcuts created for commonly used phrases or norms that can be activated with a single voice command. TalkNotes will go one step further with macros by automatically pulling patient demographic data into your customized macro.

Another option is to use the note generation products such as Quic Doc (http://www.quicdoc.com) or the ICANotes system (http://www.icanotes.com), which create documents with a few clicks on buttons to reduce text entry. Users can set up templates in which standardized text can be selected. Information from previous notes can also brought be forward to reduce additional typing. While generating the note, the program will also determine the appropriate E and M (evaluation and management) and psychotherapy codes based on the entries made.

## Electronic Medical Records

Depending on the level of sophistication necessary for medical records, physicians can use word processing documents or more sophisticated systems with built-in features such as scheduling, accounting, and billing processing. A few physicians build their own systems, using Microsoft Access to keep track of patients, medications, and visits. In essence, what you put into the system determines what you will gain from it; that is, more data entered into a structured record or data format will provide the opportunity to analyze and find more information.

There are other psychiatric patient management systems, such as Therapist Helper (http://www.helper.com), that are designed specifically for psychiatry to write therapy notes, keep track of appointments, and submit electronic billing. Other electronic medical records with a mental health component include OmniMD (http://www.omnimd.com), SQL Clinic (http://www.sqlclinic.net), and the Virtual Briefcase (http://www.thevirtualbriefcase.com). Check out what other physicians have thought about different products at EMR Update (http://www.emrupdate.com).

## Medical References

Most physicians probably will rely on traditional textbooks and pocket guides for references, but a variety of compelling resources are available on the Internet. American Psychiatric Publishing, Inc. (http://www.appi.org), provides electronic access to its journals for its subscribers. This setup permits subscribers to search for articles based on author or subject, read the articles online, and download Adobe PDF versions. In addition, if you sign up for a free Highwire account (http://highwire.stanford.edu), the abstracts of these journals can be updated to your PDA.

Medscape (http://www.medscape.com) is another popular destination for psychiatrists, offering articles and continuing medical education (CME) credits for many topics and reports from many psychiatric meetings. Ovid (http://www.ovid.com), eMedicine (http://www.emedicine.com), WebMD (http://www.webmd.com), and MD Consult (http://www.mdconsult.com) are online resources providing access to a variety of journals and textbooks on a subscription basis. Although there is an inherent value in ownership of textbooks, online subscriptions are like car leases of the newest models—

providing access to the latest in texts and journals.

In 2005, American Psychiatric Publishing, Inc., launched Psychiatry-Online (http://www.psychiatryonline.com). This new service has the complete content of DSM-IV-TR™ integrated with other essential psychiatry resources. It provides mental health professionals with comprehensive access to the many references, including DSM-IV-TR™, DSM-IV-TR™ Casebook and its Treatment Companion, and the American Psychiatric Association's Practice Guidelines for the Treatment of Psychiatric Disorders; APPI journals such as the *American Journal of Psychiatry*; textbooks including the *American Psychiatric Publishing Textbook of Clinical Psychiatry*; self-assessment tools for board certification and recertification review; CME; and news from *Psychiatric News*. A unique feature of this service is that all of the content will be linked via keywords. For example, while browsing practice guidelines, you will see links to textbook chapters and journals on that topic.

PubMed (http://www.ncbi.nlm.nih.gov/entrez/) is the gold standard site that provides for online searching of journals indexed by the Library of Medicine. Abstracts are available that can be sent to your e-mail account or printed from the computer. One of the nicely integrated features is the links to online journal access, which require you to log on to these services. If remembering your password is too difficult, allow the computer to retain **cookies**, which store this information. However, anybody with access to your computer will also have access to whatever secure Web sites for which you have enabled these cookies.

For portable medical references, Skyscape (http://www.skyscape.com), LexiComp (http://www.lexi.com), and Handheldmed (http://www.handheldmed.com) provide the majority of handheld computer-based text references. These texts are available for purchase for either the Pocket PC or Palm OS PDA, but keep in mind that the main memory of these devices may be a limitation. Fortunately, most of the texts can be stored in external memory media such as Compact Flash and Secure Digital cards.

## Continuing Medical Education

The Internet is a rich source of Web-based CME. There are many advantages associated with online CME courses, such as multimedia presentations, convenience of taking them anytime, and ability to go at your own pace. Check Medical Computing Today (http://www.medicalcomputingto-day.com/0listcme.html) for a comprehensive listing of available sites with CME for specialties. Medscape (http://www.medscape.com) is another good site for this purpose, and it also has a CME tracker once you create an account.

## Backup

Although computers are quite reliable these days, it is important for all medical providers to back up their information. Backups should be done on a daily basis at a set time such as during lunch or at the end of the day, and this process should be automated. Information can be backed up to an external removable hard drive, portable large-capacity drives such as the Iomega Zip drive, CD-RW, compact flash drives, or, for large volume, digital archive tape (DAT). One of the advantages of using rewritable media is that an archive for each day of operations can be made and recycled each week. Dantz Retrospect Backup (http://www.dantz.com) is an example of a good product with sufficient media options and speed. It will even store data online with an Internet storage provider such as XDrive (http://www.xdrive.com).

If software and data are critical to daily operations without loss of time in restoring information, a RAID (redundant array of independent disks) setup of hard drives may be needed. In this situation, the data is stored on two drives simultaneously, and if one drive fails, the other drive will automatically start to deliver the information. This level is RAID level 1 and should be set up with two drives of similar capacity. Because hard drives are available with quite large capacity yet low price per gigabyte, this setup is highly recommended. There is an excellent tutorial available at PC Tech Guide (http://www.http://www.pctechguide.com/tutorials/RAID.htm) for this setup, which is best done by those comfortable with hardware installation.

With backup and security in mind, office computers should have surge protectors to prevent data loss via power surges that may corrupt information or interfere with operation of the computer. In the event of power loss, an uninterruptible power supply (UPS) is also a must to allow time for existing data to be stored prior to computer shutdown. Notebook computer users have the advantage that their battery will provide power in the event of a power outage, but this setup will not provide emergency power to other devices such as a fax, printer, or modem. One vendor with a range of products to consider is American Power Conversion Corporation (http://www.apcc.com).

## Billing Services

Providers who see patients with insurance will benefit from sending their billing to the insurer via the computer. This service can be outsourced to a company such as BillShrinkers (http://www.billshrinkers.com) or handled by hired staff. Many vendors sell solutions that can be linked with your billing software system. Billing can be sent via a modem, or via the Internet if your office has broadband access. Having such a system will also reconcile accounts receivable in your billing software.

## Security

All providers who submit electronic billing either directly or via clearinghouses are required by the Health Information Portability and Accountability Act of 1996 (HIPAA) to guarantee security of medical information. HIPAA contains other important provisions as well, including measures specifying how and when providers may release information, requiring that they disclose to whom information is released, and holding violators accountable.

The data covered by this act is any protected health information, such as records related to a person's health, provision of care, or payment. This data includes patient identifiers, information created or received from a HIPAA covered entity, and any information electronically generated, maintained, and transmitted. A key concept to remember is that the information itself is protected, not just the record in which it appears.

The "Minimum Necessary Standard" (http://www.hhs.gov/ocr/hipaa/guidelines/minimumnecessary.pdf) states that providers must restrict protected health information disclosed to a minimum amount necessary to accomplish the purpose of disclosure. HIPAA does not specify any particular security mechanism, but it has set clear penalties for any breach of its provisions. Penalties range from $50,000 to $250,000 in fines for each occurrence as well as prison terms up to 10 years. The "minimum necessary" scope indicates that the security mechanism to be implemented must be reasonably appropriate to limit the inadvertent or unnecessary disclosure of information (http://www.cms.hhs.gov/hipaa/hipaa2/regulations/security/03–3877.pdf).

Security cannot rely solely on technology and should take into account human nature. Appropriate policies must be in place and certain protocols enacted when there is a security breach. It may not be necessary for a private practice to have a security officer, but within a group practice, someone should be designated to be in charge. Include a firm policy that any unnecessary staff access to patient information will result in dismissal. Staff and physicians should sign a security agreement affirming their understanding of this policy.

Passwords are one of the most simple yet effective mechanisms of security, but often they are forgotten or are written down and stuck on a note on the computer. Ideally, passwords should have a minimum of 6 characters, utilize a mixture of symbols and numbers, be changed on a monthly basis, and not be meaningful phrases such as the name of a pet or child. Biometric devices such as iris scanners, face recognition, and fingerprint readers are still too unreliable to be used at this time but are improving.

On the computer, any sensitive files should be encrypted for the highest level of security. No one wants to be the first physician prosecuted under HIPAA. Although this mechanism is the most secure, it can be defeated by a too-simple password used to decode the information. Another method is to use a hardware key that creates a virtual drive where data can be safely stored, such as the Bafo USB Security Key (http://www.bafo.com/bafo/productslists.asp?foproduct_id=1170) or Authenex HDLock (http://www.authenex.com/products_hdlock.cfm). Without the key and password, there is no access to the data. Ideally, there should also be a tracking program that logs everyone who uses the computer, when each one used it, and which files were accessed. Any changes to the medical record must be recorded so that any attempts to modify data are also known. When the user leaves the computer, the user should log off manually or be automatically logged off so that no one else can use his or her access level.

Computers connected to the Internet should utilize firewall software. These programs track when outside programs attempt to send information to and gain information from the computer from the different **ports**. By designating which programs are allowed to connect to the Internet, one can prevent unauthorized intrusions. Some popular firewall programs are ZoneAlarm, Norton Internet Security, and Tiny Personal Firewall.

Hardware security can be accomplished with wire cables or a security plate to lock the computer to a desk. Vulnerable peripherals such as ZIP drives, small scanners, and tape drives, which may contain sensitive data, should also be secured. An alternative to using hardware security is to use Internet-based data backup such as IBackup (http://www.iback.up.com). One of the advantages of Internet backup is that the data are safely stored in a remote location in the event of a theft or even a fire.

# ▍ CONNECTIVITY

## Remote Access

When you are away from the office, say at a meeting, and need access to your data, there are several methods you can use to connect to your computer. If your desktop and notebook computer have Windows XP, there is a built-in remote assistance program that permits control over your computer over the Internet. It is a simple matter of sending a permission file to access the computer via e-mail. You can send one to yourself by making an online Web account for e-mail. Once you have an Internet connection on the remote computer, you can then access your office computer. Other methods include using software products such as PCAnywhere (http://www.symantec.com) or Laplink (http://www.laplink.com), or a service provider such as GoToMyPC (http://www.gotomypc.com).

## Telemedicine

Telemedicine typically refers to video conferencing as a method for "visiting" a patient, but actually telemedicine spans a variety of methods such as e-mail, instant messaging, and traditional telephone calls. There are many issues limiting the practice of video conferencing, such as reimbursement by insurance, practicing across state lines, sufficient bandwidth for quality of session, safety issues in case of emergencies, and costs of the hardware and software. Telemedicine using videoconferencing is advantageous for practitioners with patients in rural settings far away, but the available connection speed is often limited.

E-mail is a great way to communicate with your patients and with other professionals. Many providers are somewhat leery of this communication method because of fears about liability, security, time requirements, and reimbursements. If you plan to use e-mail with your patients, you should make arrangements regarding what issues e-mail can be used for, security methods such as encryption, type of urgency allowable, and assurances that only you or your nurse are reading the messages. One method to ensure secure communications with your patients is to use the Medem Secure Messaging and Online Consultation services (http://www.medem.com/phy/phy_faq_physician.cfm). Always use a professional e-mail account separately from a private or home account to avoid a mix-up. A great resource regarding e-mail communication is the "Guidelines for the Clinical Use of Electronic Mail with Patients" published by Kane and Sands (1998) in the *Journal of the American Medical Informatics Association*.

A key issue with e-mail is that there are two types of systems, Web-based and client-server. In a client-server model, the desktop computer will download the e-mail, and responses and new messages are sent back through the server. Typically, these are **POP** (post office protocol) e-mail accounts provided by your ISP setup with certain e-mail clients such as Outlook Express or Eudora. In contrast, the advantage of a Web-based e-mail account is that all messages are kept on the server, and access requires only a Web browser and an Internet connection. However, with Web-based systems there will be a limit on storage, which limits the ability to save e-mail for reference later.

The best plan is to have a client-server account but to access it via a service such as Mail2Web (http://www.mail2web.com). In this manner, while you are away at a meeting, you can check your e-mail that normally would be downloaded to your client software. Messages sent will appear as if you were using your account from home and will only have a small tag at the end of the message highlighting the service. Later when you return home, you can download those messages onto your hard disk. In addition, many ISPs such as Earthlink (http://www.earthlink.com) offer a Web-mail-based system that works with your regular client-server account. Some cellular phones have wireless application protocol (**WAP**) that will enable you to check your e-mail as well.

Some providers are beginning to use instant messaging (**IM**) to conduct therapy with their patients online. In situations where telephone calls are prohibitively expensive, IM is a great alternative if both parties have a fast enough Internet connection. This type of contact is not unlike a phone conversation because it is conducted in real time. However, the popular instant messaging clients are too insecure for sensitive conversations because all data is routed unencrypted through the central server. There are enterprise-level products to secure IM traffic, but products available to individual users to encrypt communication are Secure Shuttle Transport (http://www.secureshuttle.com), DBabble (http://free.dbabble.com), and PSST (http://www.psst.sourceforge.net).

The advantage of IM over e-mail for therapy with patients is that it is a one-on-one dialogue that will not have the distraction of other messages showing up in the e-mail queue. It is possible to include other parties if desired, and the multimedia features such as voice and video may provide additional cues about the interaction. Because it is a direct channel of communication with visual references to previous dialogue, IM creates an environment of an active conversation. One of the detractions is that the speed of the conversation is typically limited by the typing speed of the participants. Using voice overcomes this limitation, but it should not be used unless the Internet connection is sufficiently fast via broadband, such as over a cable modem or DSL.

# ▮ CONCLUSION

It is nearly impossible in today's medical practice to not have a computer in the office. Computers provide a rich and readily available resource of reference information, a medium for communication via e-mail or instant messaging, a method for documentation and billing, and a source for continuing education. The rapid development of new hardware and software may cause anxiety that today's purchase is already obsolete; however, the time-saving benefits are significant and outweigh that issue. The ideas described in this chapter have offered an overview and a starting point for your technological decision making. You may wish to consider joining a group of fellow psychiatrists such as the American Association for Technology in Psychiatry (http://www.techpsych.org) to learn novel methods by which technology plays a role in providing patient care.

## ▮ REFERENCE

Kane B, Sands DZ: Guidelines for the clinical use of electronic mail with patients. J Am Med Inform Assoc 5:104–111, 1998

# Glossary

**Bandwidth.**   The capacity of a communications channel to send information over time, measured in bits per second (bps). DSL and cable modems are considered to have relatively high bandwidth compared with dial-up modems.

**Broadband.**   A communication network in which the bandwidth can be divided and shared by multiple simultaneous signals (voice, data, video). Typically refers to Internet access at high speeds such as that provided by DSL and cable modem.

**Cable modem.**   A service that provides fast Internet access over the cable television network coaxial cable. Typically provides fast service but is shared among a number of users. It will slow down if there are many users on concurrently.

**Client.**   An element of client-server architecture. It is a program on a computer that relies on a connection to a server computer to perform some operations. For example, an e-mail client is an application that enables you to send and receive e-mail on a server.

**Domain name.**   The text name that links to the numerical Internet protocol (IP) number or address of a Web site; in the example *domain.net*, the domain name refers to the IP address 123.123.25.25. Domain names are easier to remember than the numerical address and must be registered with a domain name registrar such as Registrar.com.

**Domain name registration.**   The process of registering a domain name with a specific IP address in the domain name database, done by a domain name registration company.

**DSL (digital subscriber line).**    A service that provides fast Internet access over a regular copper phone line at varying downstream speeds. Typically, the speed from the Internet service provider to the computer will depend on the distance from the central office and other factors. An advantage over cable modem is that the download speed is dedicated and not shared.

**Dynamic IP address.**    An IP address that changes each time your computer reconnects to the Internet service provider (ISP). A dynamic IP address is cheaper than a static IP and is best for most general uses. *See* **Static IP address.**

**Firewall.**    Hardware and/or software used between internal local area networks (LANs) and the Internet for protection. A firewall allows only specific kinds of messages from the Internet to flow in and out of the internal network so as to prevent intruders or hackers from using the Internet to break into the system.

**HTML (hypertext markup language).**    The coding language used to create hypertext documents for use on the Internet. It contains a set of codes inserted in a file that tells the Web browser how to display a Web page's words and images for viewing and linking.

**IM (instant messaging).**    A service that alerts users when friends or colleagues are online and allows them to communicate with each other in private online chat areas. This service requires that both users have the same IM client.

**IP (Internet protocol).**    The communications protocol underlying the Internet, which allows networks of computers to communicate with each other quickly over a variety of physical links.

**IP address.**    The numerical address by which a location on the Internet is identified. Computers on the Internet use IP addresses to route information and establish connections among themselves. People in general use the much easier to remember names made possible by the Domain Name System.

**ISDN (integrated services digital network).**    A digital telephony method that allows connections to the Internet over standard phone lines at higher speeds than a 56K modem, but that requires a specialized phone line. Nowadays it is becoming less popular with the development of DSL and cable modem.

**ISP (Internet service provider).**    The company that provides the Internet connection to your computer. This service will give your computer an IP address, which may be either *dynamic* or *static.*

**Javascript.**   A scripting language that performs certain functions on a Web site to make it more interactive. For example, it can display forms and buttons or make special mouse pointers appear.

**Kiosk.**   A computer in specialized and strong housing that is placed where people can use it to find information, or conduct transactions.

**LAN (local area network).**   A network of computers interconnected via wire or wireless.

**MAC (media access control).**   The globally unique hardware address of an Ethernet network interface card or wireless access card. Used to limit access to a router for Internet access.

**PDA (personal digital assistant).**   A small device used to organize personal information such as notes, calendar, and addresses, as well as to access other medical resources such as medical textbooks, drug information, etc.

**PDF (portable document format).**   A file format created by Adobe that maintains the layout of the original document. Popular for distributing documents on the Internet. The free version of Adobe Acrobat Reader allows computers to read the document without having the software that created it.

**POP (post office protocol).**   A protocol designed to allow users to transmit stored mail from the server to the local mailbox on the client machine after the user is authenticated.

**Port.**   The name given to an endpoint of an IP connection on a LAN or on the Internet. For example, port 80 is where HTTP data is transmitted. Also the name of a physical connective device (such as a parallel port for printers).

**Router.**   A hardware device or software in a computer that directs information packets to the next point toward their destination between at least two computer networks. A typical example is the connection between an office LAN and the Internet.

**Server.**   A central computer that manages users, computers, settings, and applications as well as resources such as files, printers, or even the Internet access.

**SSID (service set identifier).** The network name that identifies a wireless network; broadcast by the wireless access point. Ideally, to make finding the network more difficult for intruders, the wireless access point should *not* broadcast the SSID.

**Static IP address.** An IP address that always remains the same for your Internet connection. A static IP address is necessary if your office computer is your Web site server and your IP address is registered with a domain name. *See* **Dynamic IP address.**

**URL (uniform resource locator).** The distinct address that identifies a resource on the Internet such as a Web site. An example of a URL is <http://www.appi.org>.

**WAP (wireless application protocol).** The worldwide standard developed by the WAP forum for providing Internet communications and other advanced telephony services on digital mobile phones, pagers, and personal digital assistants.

**Web hosting.** This service permits storage of a Web site's HTML documents and related files on a Web server on the Internet for viewing. Also known as *site hosting.*

**WEP (wired equivalent privacy).** An encryption system that encrypts data on 802.11b wireless networks. The encrypted data can be read only by authorized users with the correct decryption key. (The 802.11b standard is a set of specifications for wireless systems established by the Institute of Electrical and Electronics Engineers [IEEE].)

**Wi-Fi (wireless fidelity).** Another name for the IEEE 802.11b wireless protocol standard. It is a trade name marketed by the Wireless Ethernet Compatibility Alliance (WECA). WECA-certified products are interoperable with each other even if they are from different manufacturers.

**Wireless access point.** A device that provides or hosts wireless Internet access to computers with wireless network adapters.

**Wireless repeater.** A device that extends the range of a wireless Internet access signal by boosting the signal strength.

# 8

# HOW TO COLLABORATE WITH PRIMARY CARE PHYSICIANS TO ACHIEVE BETTER OUTCOMES

*Steven Cole, M.D.*

In 1993, the Epidemiologic Catchment Area study (ECA) revealed that 28% of Americans experience significant mental disorders at some time in their lives, yet about half of these individuals never get any mental health treatment (Regier et al. 1993). In a surprising finding, the authors of that study discovered and named the "de facto mental health" delivery system in the primary care sector. That is, they found that more Americans were being treated for mental disorders in the primary health care sector than by behavioral health specialists. In 1993, 41% of all antidepressant medication visits were to primary care physicians (vs. 44% to psychiatrists) (Pincus et al. 1998). By 1998, 50% of all antidepressants were being prescribed by primary care physicians (Sleath and Shih 2003), and by 2003, this figure approached 70% (personal communication, pharmaceutical industry sources). A matter of related interest is that the total number of people treated for depression in the United States almost tripled between 1987 and 1997 (Olfson et al. 2002).

The recognition of this de facto mental health system has led to reasonable concerns about the quality and outcomes of care for the treatment of mental health problems in primary care. There are now numerous studies documenting inadequate recognition and treatment of depression in primary care, as well as suboptimal outcomes (Cole 2001; Cole and Bird 2000). These problems have led to efforts to improve the mental health training of primary care physicians (Gerrity et al. 1999) as well as efforts to improve the integration of primary care with behavioral health specialty care (Cole and Raju 1996). The best outcomes documented for depression and anxiety disorders in primary care have resulted from the implementation of new "collaborative care" or "disease management" models of care (Badamgarav et al. 2003; Katon et al. 1995; Oxman et al. 2002; Roy-Byrne et al. 2001).

Collaborative or disease management care of depression in primary care includes many elements, ranging from improved patient and physician education to better monitoring and tracking of patient progress and care coordination, but all models include improved integration of behavioral health specialty care with primary care and improved communication. Thus, the future of psychiatry with respect to mental disorders in primary care will move from a "de facto" mental health system in primary care to one of explicit partnership. In this chapter, I review the most common mental disorders in primary care, discuss common barriers to improved mental health care in primary care, summarize evidence-based models for improved collaboration, and present suggestions for junior psychiatrists on ways they can improve their own interaction with primary care physicians.

## ∎ COMMON PSYCHIATRIC DISORDERS IN PRIMARY CARE

The four most prominent groups of psychiatric disorders presenting in primary care are affective, anxiety, substance abuse, and somatoform disorders. Approximately 25%–50% of all attendees at primary care outpatient clinics have one or more of these disorders. Primary care physicians often find these patients to be complex (Cole 2001), "difficult" (Hahn et al. 1996), and even at times "hateful" (Groves 1978). Recognition and treatment of the disorder is often problematic.

## ∎ TEN BARRIERS TO INTEGRATION OF CARE

Ten barriers to improved recognition and management of these common psychiatric disorders have been identified (Cole and Raju 1996). These include 1) the biomedical culture of general medical practice; 2) the stigma of mental disorders; 3) the "fallacy of good reasons" (explaining away a psychiatric disorder as "expected"); 4) the fear of opening Pandora's box (avoiding emotional problems for fear of being overwhelmed); 5) somatization (the tendency of patient and physician to focus on physical manifestations of psychiatric disorders); 6) financial disincentives (lack of reimbursement); 7) administrative and social barriers; 8) insufficient knowledge; 9) insufficient skills; and 10) avoidance from habit. Overcoming these problems require interventions on many levels, but there is now increasing evidence that the barriers can be overcome by a concerted collaborative approach, as described below.

# ▌ THREE TYPES OF CLINICAL INTEGRATION: REFERRAL, CONSULTATION, AND COLLABORATION

New models of collaboration and integration have been clarified, and there is now a robust evidence base for them. There are three main types of coordination of care between psychiatrists and primary care physicians: referral, consultation, and collaboration (or co-management). *Referral* of patients from primary care to psychiatry refers to the transfer of care and clinical responsibility from the primary care physician to the psychiatrist. Referrals based on this traditional model will certainly persist in the future but will decrease in frequency relative to newer models. *Consultation* refers to the one-time assessment of a patient by a psychiatrist, with care continued by the primary care clinician. One-time consultations will certainly continue in the future, but they have not been shown to have a dramatic effect on ultimate outcome (Levenson et al. 1992), and they too will decrease proportionately. *Collaboration* or *co-management* has been shown to dramatically improve outcomes and will increase sharply in the next decade. It will be important for the psychiatrist of the future to understand these different models of integration and develop clinical integration skills appropriate to each.

# ▌ EVIDENCE BASE FOR COLLABORATIVE CARE

In 1993, only 3% of patients with mental health problems reported receiving mental health care from both primary care physicians and behavioral health specialists (Regier et al. 1993). With the emergent and increasing evidence base for collaborative models of care, it is reasonable to expect this proportion to rise dramatically in the next decade. Beginning with the seminal contribution of Katon et al. in 1995, a generation of studies has demonstrated that systematic integration of behavioral health care specialists, along with care coordination of patients, leads to improved response rates of depression. In general, collaborative care leads to rates of response ranging from 60% to 80%—compared with response rates in "care as usual" by the primary care physician in the range of 50%—even after 1 year (Oxman et al. 2002).

## ∎ EFFECTIVE COMMUNICATION WITH PRIMARY CARE PHYSICIANS

On an individual level, what can the junior psychiatrist do to improve the chances of positive interactions with primary care physicians? The first step in developing positive interactions is mastery of effective communication behaviors. From an educational or self-development point of view, this goal can be addressed by considering the domains of knowledge, attitudes, and skills.

## ∎ KNOWLEDGE: THREE RULES OF EFFECTIVE COMMUNICATION

There are three cardinal rules of communication between psychiatrists and primary care physicians: 1) communicate, 2) communicate briefly, and 3) communicate in English. The first rule of effective communication is "communicate." This, of course, seems obvious, but it is not. The single most important and compelling criticism of psychiatrists by primary care physicians is the common refrain "psychiatrists *never* communicate with me about my patients, once I have referred them for an evaluation." I often challenge the physicians from whom I have heard these comments, saying something like, "I am sure you do not mean they *never* communicate. You probably mean they *hardly* ever communicate." The primary care physicians usually respond, in effect, "No, you heard me correctly…I *never* hear back from psychiatrists."

So, let it be clearly understood: Because primary care physicians have made it clear that they want to hear feedback from psychiatrists, the first cardinal rule of effective communication is "communicate."

The second cardinal rule of effective communication is "communicate briefly." When psychiatrists do communicate with primary care physicians, sometimes the communication is too lengthy, too detailed, and lacking in focus. Because psychiatrists are usually trained to elicit a broad range of psychosocial data that may affect a mental disorder, and sometimes this information is complex, psychiatrists have a tendency to describe these details too extensively. This overloads primary care physicians who do want to hear information, but to hear it in a form that is easily assimilated.

The third rule of effective communication is "communicate in English." When psychiatrists communicate, they sometimes understand the psychosocial information they obtain in terms of psychological concepts unfamiliar to primary care physicians. "Defense mechanisms," "cognitive distortions," and the like are not concepts that primary care physicians utilize in everyday clinical care. The psychiatrist should not tell a primary care physician, for example, that his or her patient is "suffering from a negative maternal introject," or that the patient is frustrating for the physician because of unresolved transference or countertransference issues in the relationship. Communication must be simple, direct, and clinically relevant, with information expressed in understandable terms.

# ▌ ATTITUDES

Maladaptive attitudes often dominate negative interactions between psychiatrists and primary care physicians—often at the house staff level during training years, as well as afterwards in the community. The following maladaptive attitudes on the part of psychiatrists inhibit effective relationships: 1) primary care physicians are not interested in psychosocial issues; 2) primary care physicians do not want to hear from me/do not have the time to hear from me; and 3) primary care physicians do not consider psychiatrists "real" doctors. Each of these is false.

Many psychiatrists hold the self-justifying impression that they alone represent the major "caring" profession among the medical specialties. This can lead to a defensive or aggressive posture toward medical colleagues, based on the assumption that other physicians do not "care" about the emotional dimensions of patient care the way psychiatrists do. It is important for psychiatrists to realize that they do not hold any special claim on caring. Primary care physicians do, in fact, take care of their patients and do, in fact, emotionally care for their patients as well. Because they care emotionally for their patients, they generally do want to hear from psychiatrists, particularly if the information provided can be useful for patient care. Finally, psychiatrists sometimes also take the defensive position that primary care physicians do not see them as "real" doctors. For the most part, this is also incorrect.

I encourage young psychiatrists to assume that primary care physicians do care about their patients, do want to hear (albeit in short, understandable terms) about their patients, and do treat psychiatrists as genuine colleagues who can contribute to care of patients.

# ∎ SKILLS: THREE FUNCTIONS OF EFFECTIVE COMMUNICATION

Following a communication skills model developed for doctor-patient communication (Cole et al. 2000), I propose that young psychiatrists think of skills development for their relationships with primary care physicians across the three functions of effective communication. The functions are the same for colleagues as they are for patients: gather data, develop rapport (respond to emotions), and educate.

## #1: Gather Data From the Referring Physician

It is important to determine what the referring physician wants from the psychiatric evaluation. The written referral may be helpful, but more often than not, the information provided in a written referral is nonspecific, such as "see and evaluate." The psychiatrist is often uncertain whether the referring physician is interested in transferring care to the psychiatrist or wants a one-time consultation. The reason for a referral may be to evaluate substance abuse or domestic violence—and without information from the referring physician, the psychiatrist may conduct an entire evaluation without any awareness of the real reason, if the patient is not forthcoming with this information. A direct contact (preferably by telephone) with the referring physician *before* the psychiatric evaluation can be time-saving in the final analysis and can lead to more effective care for the patient and better relationships with the primary care physician.

## #2: Develop Rapport and Respond to the Primary Care Physician's Emotions

Just as rapport and response to patient emotions are central to patient care, rapport and appropriate response to the primary care physician's emotions are central to effective relationships with colleagues. Psychiatric patients are often "difficult" or even "hateful," and the psychiatrist can improve his or her relationships with referring physicians by acknowledging these difficulties directly. In hearing about a difficult patient or even after evaluating a difficult patient, the psychiatrist can build rapport with a referring primary care physician with *empathic* comments such as, "It sounds like this is certainly a difficult case," or "I can understand how this patient is very troubling." If the referring physician has already begun some treatment, it is important to *respect* these interventions. Comments such as, "I understand why you chose to initiate this particular treatment intervention with the patient…I think I would recommend the following adjustments…" can be very reassuring. Finally, the psychiatrist should offer *support* for the referring physician with comments such as, "I will do the best I can to help you with this difficult patient…"

## #3: Educate the Referring Physician

The third function for effective communication with referring physicians is the same as the third function for effective communication with patients: educate. Just as patients must understand their illness and its treatment for effective management, referring physicians need to understand the problems of their patients. Physicians must use focused, clear language that is understandable and usable by their patients. Psychiatrists must use focused, clear language that is understandable and usable by their consultees. Psychiatrists should be succinct and practical when educating primary care physicians. Referring primary care physicians want to know the diagnosis and the treatment recommendations. The most important skill for good education involves use of *simple, direct, focused statements.* Psychiatrists should tell the referring physician the diagnosis ("I think your patient has major depression") and treatment recommendations ("The medication you started is fine, but I doubled the dose because the patient has not yet reached full remission").

In terms of education, referring primary care physicians usually want to know what they can do for the patient. *Do not tell the referring primary care physician to "be supportive."* This is an insulting and meaningless recommendation because it implies that the primary care physician may not already be supportive to his or her patient, and it also is so grossly general that it renders meaningless the true value and potential of the primary care physician's collaborative intervention. Instead of the generalization "be supportive," or "offer support," the psychiatrist should focus on some specific and relevant psychosocial interventions that are, in fact, practical for the primary care physician and that will be helpful for the patient. For example, a specific recommendation could be something like the following:

> "While the patient is still recovering from the depression, I think it would be helpful for you to see him for his diabetes every month, until the depression is resolved, and listen for just a minute or two at least about his current problems at home. You don't need to get into a lot of specific detail or spend a lot of time on this, but the patient's current marital distress feeds into his depression and will make diabetic control more difficult."

All three functions—gathering data, responding to emotions, and educating—should be attended to in *every* communication with the referring primary care physician. Although this might at first seem too complex and time-consuming, neglecting one of the three functions can lead to ineffective and unsatisfactory relationships with sources of referral and also to ineffective patient care. In general, these communications do not need to take a great deal of time, even if all three functions are addressed. In general, I aim to complete the focused communication in about three minutes and offer more detailed communication only if the referring physician asks for further information and clarification.

## ∎ THE WRITTEN COMMUNICATION

Just as focus and brevity are essential for the verbal communication, written communication with referring primary care physicians must be succinct and clear. The more closely psychiatrists follow the style and formal (and informal) conventions of their medical colleagues, the more likely it is that the psychiatrists will be seen as physicians and the more likely it is that their patients will be seen as true medical patients (Cohen-Cole 1989).

*The assessment and recommendations should appear at the very front of the consultation report, and they should be numbered.* Psychiatrists are the only physicians who seem to write full text paragraphs for their assessments and recommendations. I think this is often a reflection of unfocused, rambling thinking. *In communications with primary care physicians, do not write five-axis diagnoses.* Primary care physicians simply do not think in terms of five axes. For assessment purposes, they do not make distinctions between Axis I and Axis II; they are already aware of Axis III issues; and information they might find useful that is captured in Axis IV and Axis V can be summarized for them in the database. When psychiatrists write five-axis diagnoses, they reinforce the idea that psychiatrists and their patients are different from other physicians and patients and that they communicate about patients in bizarre conventions that do not apply to other medical patients.

The database should be similarly focused and succinct, covering essential elements of the history of present illness, relevant past history and social history, and focused mental status examination. *When reporting the mental status examination, do not write a paragraph.* When psychiatrists write a narrative paragraph describing the mental status examination results, they again reinforce the idea that psychiatrists and their patients are different from other doctors and patients. The mental status examination is the objective part of the psychiatric examination, and format and presentation should correspond to the way a physical examination is recorded by physicians. In fact, the mental status exam is a part of the overall examination of the patient for all physicians. Authoritative interviewing texts usually place the mental status examination as part of the neurological examination for recording and data entry purposes. I recommend a six-element mental status examination that is recorded in separate bullet points, as the abdominal and cardiac exams are separated by bullets. These are the core mental status elements that should be included in the basic consultation report (Cole et al. 2000):

1. General description
2. Speech
3. Mood/affect
4. Thought (including suicidal/homicidal ideation and hallucinations/delusions)
5. Cognition/sensorium
6. Insight/judgment

The following is an example of a brief written mental status examination report that would be useful to primary care physicians:

1. General description: 60-year-old male, well dressed, good grooming
2. Speech: Very slow; little spontaneity; not slurred; goal directed and organized
3. Mood/affect: Reports being "sad"; patient tearful during interview
4. Thought: Patient wants to feel "better"; no evidence of psychosis; no evidence of suicidality or dangerousness to others
5. Cognition/sensorium: Patient is oriented in all spheres; remembers 3/3 objects in 3 minutes; spells "world" backwards without error
6. Insight/judgment: Good—understands that he is depressed and needs treatment

# ▌ CONCLUSION

Collaboration with medical colleagues is an important part of psychiatric practice. Learning basic principles for effective communication and developing appropriate attitudes and effective verbal and written skills for collaboration are important for good patient care and for maintaining satisfying professional and business relationships with medical colleagues.

# ∎ REFERENCES

Badamgarav E, Weingarten SR, Henning JM, et al: Effectiveness of disease management programs in depression: a systematic review. Am J Psychiatry 160:2080–2090, 2003

Cohen-Cole S: A Practical Guide to Performing the Consultation. Philadelphia, PA, Lippincott, 1989

Cole S[A]: Mental and Behavioral Disorders in Primary Care: Bridging the Gap. St. Louis, MO, Mosby-Yearbook, 2001

Cole SA, Bird J: The Medical Interview: The Three-Function Approach, 2nd Edition. St. Louis, MO, Mosby-Yearbook, 2000

Cole SA, Raju M: Overcoming barriers to integration of primary care and behavioral healthcare: focus on knowledge and skills. Behav Healthc Tomorrow 5(5):30–37, 1996

Cole S[A], Raju M, Dietrich A, et al: The MacArthur Foundation Depression Education Program for Primary Care Physicians: rationale, participants' workbook, and facilitators' guide. Gen Hosp Psychiatry 22:299–358, 2000

Gerrity MS, Cole SA, Dietrich AJ, et al: Improving the recognition and management of depression: is there a role for physician education? J Fam Pract 48:949–957, 1999

Groves JE: Taking care of the hateful patient. N Engl J Med 298:883–887, 1978

Hahn SR, Kroenke K, Spitzer RL, et al: The difficult patient: prevalence, psychopathology, and functional impairment. J Gen Intern Med 11:1–8 [erratum, 11:191], 1996

Katon W, Von Korff M, Lin E, et al: Collaborative management to achieve treatment guidelines: impact on depression in primary care. JAMA 273:1026–1031, 1995

Levenson JL, Hamer RM, Rossiter LF: A randomized controlled study of psychiatric consultation guided by screening in general medical inpatients. Am J Psychiatry 149:631–637, 1992

Olfson M, Marcus SC, Weissman MM, et al: National trends in the use of psychotropic medications by children. J Am Acad Child Adolesc Psychiatry 41:514–521, 2002

Oxman TE, Dietrich AJ, Williams JW Jr, et al: A three-component model for re-engineering systems for the treatment of depression in primary care. Psychosomatics 43:441–450, 2002

Pincus HA, Tanielian TL, Marcus SC, et al: Prescribing trends in psychotropic medications: primary care, psychiatry, and other medical specialties. JAMA 279:526–531, 1998

Regier DA, Narrow WE, Rae DS, et al: The de facto US mental and addictive disorders service system: Epidemiologic Catchment Area prospective 1-year prevalence rates of disorders and services. Arch Gen Psychiatry 50:85–94, 1993

Roy-Byrne PP, Katon W, Cowley DS, et al: A randomized effectiveness trial of collaborative care for patients with panic disorder in primary care. Arch Gen Psychiatry 58:869–876, 2001

Sleath B, Shih YC: Sociological influences on antidepressant prescribing. Soc Sci Med 56:1335–1344, 2003

# 9

# TOP TEN LEGAL AND RISK MANAGEMENT AREAS OF CONCERN FOR PSYCHIATRISTS

*Anne Marie "Nancy" Wheeler, J.D.*

Most psychiatrists spend several intense years in medical school and residency training in order to practice psychiatry, not law. More than a few psychiatrists have expressed to this author a strong desire to stay as far away from the courtroom as possible. However, it is impossible to navigate a psychiatric practice in today's world without some familiarity with legal and risk management issues.

This chapter is an attempt to explain, in layman's terms, the top legal issues of concern for psychiatrists in the twenty-first century. It is not designed to burden the psychiatrist with a second career in law. Rather, the chapter is written to help the practicing psychiatrist spot issues of concern and act proactively to prevent legal problems before it's too late.

---

DISCLAIMER: This chapter is intended solely to provide general information on medical legal issues. It is not intended to constitute legal advice. Legal counsel should be consulted for specific advice.

# ∎ THE TOP TEN LEGAL ISSUES FOR PSYCHIATRISTS

## #1: Establishing Practice Rules and Boundaries With Patients

Many lawsuits, licensure board complaints, and complaints to association ethics bodies arise as a result of misunderstandings between psychiatrists and their patients. One way to avoid such complaints is to establish clear boundaries and practice parameters at the outset of treatment. A growing trend among psychiatrists today is the use of a fact sheet, a patient brochure, or some type of document that sets forth an understanding between psychiatrist and patient. In essence, this document is a type of informed consent that clarifies the expectations of both parties. The following list encompasses many issues that are often included in such a document:

- Psychiatrist's credentials
- Approach or theoretical orientation
- Medical and financial record issues, including name and number of records custodian in event of psychiatrist's death or disability
- Risks and benefits of treatment (separate and specific informed consent documents that confirm the discussion of risks and benefits of a certain medication, psychotherapy, or other treatment, and that are signed by the patient, may be indicated in certain circumstances or jurisdictions)
- Financial issues, including
  —fees and charges
  —insurance and managed care participation
  —responsibility for payment
- Cancellation of appointments and related charges
- Whether supervision or consultation is obtained from other professionals
- Resolutions of disputes/complaints
- Confidentiality, privilege, and privacy (this information may now be included in a HIPAA Notice of Privacy Practices; see discussion in next section)

## #2: Confidentiality, Privilege, and HIPAA Privacy

*Confidentiality* refers to the ethical duty on the part of psychiatrists to refrain from disclosing information learned from their patients. The duty has its roots in the Hippocratic Oath. In modern times, this ethical duty has developed into a legal duty, the breach of which may lead to damages in a civil lawsuit.

*Privilege* is a legal term of art and typically is embodied in state statutes or rules of evidence. Ordinarily, privilege is invoked in the context of a legal proceeding. The patient (or his legal representative), not the psychiatrist, is the "holder" of the privilege. As such, the patient is the one who claims or waives the privilege. Privilege statutes often are riddled with exceptions. For example, privilege in some states may be waived automatically when a patient puts his or her emotional condition into issue in a lawsuit. The concept of privilege has been extended in recent years to certain cases in federal court (Jaffee v. Redmond 1996).

*Privacy* is a term that refers to the right of a person to be left alone and free from unwanted intrusions. It has often been used interchangeably with the concepts of confidentiality and privilege. Since the advent of the HIPAA Privacy Rule, the concept of privacy has been broadened to encompass certain patient rights, such as the right to access one's medical information and the right to amend one's record.

What is HIPAA and how does it affect the practice of psychiatry? "HIPAA" is the acronym for the Health Insurance Portability and Accountability Act of 1996 (Pub. L. No. 104–191). One part of this broad law is entitled "Administration Simplification"; it calls for standards governing transactions and code sets, unique identifiers, security, and privacy of health care information. Implementing regulations dealing with privacy of health care information were issued in December 2000, and a second (final) version was published in August 2002 (45 CFR § 160.101 et seq.). They are commonly referred to as the HIPAA *Privacy Rule*.

The Privacy Rule applies to any "covered entity," which includes health care providers who engage in at least one electronic transaction for which the Secretary of Health and Human Services has adopted a standard. If a psychiatrist submits claims electronically or hires a billing service to perform such tasks on his behalf, the psychiatrist is most likely a covered entity who must comply with the HIPAA regulations. If a psychiatrist does not engage in any insurance reimbursement and does not conduct any transactions electronically (i.e., submits all insurance claims, etc., on paper), he or she will likely not be considered a covered entity (Centers for Medicare and Medicaid Services ["CMS"] 2004). However, even a psychiatrist who does not technically have to comply with the Rule should be aware that current standards regarding privacy, confidentiality, and client rights (such as right to access records) will likely be influenced by HIPAA requirements.

Any psychiatrist covered by HIPAA should have come into compliance with the Privacy Rule by April 14, 2003. Any covered psychiatrist who is not yet compliant with HIPAA, or any psychiatrist just starting out in private practice, will need to appoint a privacy officer. (The privacy officer may be the psychiatrist or the office manager in a small psychiatric practice.) He or she will then wish to gather all policies, fact sheets, disclosure statements, informed consent forms, and so forth that have any bearing on issues of confidentiality, privacy, and the release of information and records. The psychiatrist will need to begin the process of evaluating these policies and documents to ensure that they match HIPAA's requirements, including those regarding mandated notice to clients of the potential uses and disclosures that may be made of their protected health information. Furthermore, policies related to client access to records, amendment of records, and accounting of disclosures must be evaluated or created in response to HIPAA. The psychiatrist may also need to revise the "authorization" forms used to release information to third parties. In addition, the psychiatrist must provide training to staff, if applicable, on his or her established privacy practices.

"Psychotherapy notes" are given special protection under HIPAA. The definition of psychotherapy notes in the HIPAA Privacy Rule is as follows: "notes recorded (in any medium) by a health care provider who is a mental health professional documenting or analyzing the contents of conversation during a private counseling session or a group, joint, or family counseling session and that are separated from the rest of the individual's medical record" (45 CFR § 164.501). The definition does not include such items as counseling session start and stop times, diagnosis, treatment plan, prognosis, and progress to date. The HIPAA regulations require specific "authorization" to release psychotherapy notes. Psychiatrists who are covered by HIPAA will need to assess whether they will separate "psychotherapy notes" from the rest of the information recorded, thus keeping two sets of records. Although this dual notekeeping practice is not mandated by the Privacy Rule, some patients may expect that their psychotherapy notes will be protected by HIPAA.

The drafters of HIPAA envisioned it as providing a "floor level" of privacy. Generally, HIPAA will not preempt state laws governing confidentiality and privacy unless those state laws are contrary to HIPAA. If a state law is more stringent, or provides greater protection of the patient's rights, the state law may apply. Some states and professional organizations have engaged in analyses regarding whether state law or HIPAA will apply in certain situations. The Health Privacy Project's Web site also contains a number of state law summaries (Health Privacy Project 2004).

If a covered psychiatrist enters into any agreements with outside vendors or consultants (e.g., billing services, attorneys, accountants) with whom he or she shares protected health information, the psychiatrist should have a "business associate contract" that describes how each contractor will protect the health care information. The agreements should also limit particular uses and disclosures of information. Model business associate contract provisions are available on the Web site of the Office for Civil Rights, United States Department of Health and Human Services (Office for Civil Rights 2002).

The American Psychiatric Association (APA) has developed certain templates and other materials addressing the HIPAA privacy concerns of psychiatrists. These templates include the required "Notice of Privacy Practices" and business associate contract language. Information is available to members on the APA Web site (American Psychiatric Association 2004). The Health Privacy Project site (see the reference list in this chapter) and various medical and mental health organizations also have useful Web sites. Information on small group practices is available through the Workgroup for Electronic Data Interchange (WEDI) (Workgroup for Electronic Data Interchange 2004). Furthermore, one may access the text of the regulations and other helpful information on the HIPAA Web site of the Office for Civil Rights, Department of Health and Human Services (Office for Civil Rights 2004).

One of the most common legal issues that creates anxiety for today's practicing psychiatrist is how to handle a subpoena. HIPAA has added another level of complexity to this frequently encountered issue. The Privacy Rule *permits* a psychiatrist to disclose information in response to a subpoena if he or she receives "satisfactory assurance" from the party who sent the subpoena that reasonable efforts have been made to ensure that the patient has been given notice of the request. Furthermore, the psychiatrist may also turn over information in response to a subpoena if he or she receives "satisfactory assurance" that efforts have been made to secure a "qualified protective order."[1]

However, if the psychiatrist keeps "psychotherapy notes" as defined by HIPAA, those notes should not be released without specific patient authorization. Additionally, as mentioned earlier, if state law imposes conditions that are more protective of patient privacy than HIPAA, state law will apply. Furthermore, even if HIPAA *permits* a psychiatrist to release records as set forth here, the psychiatrist should make every effort to protect the patient's confidential information. Because of the complexities that HIPAA has introduced, the following are guidelines for a psychiatrist who must respond to a subpoena:

---

[1]A "qualified protective order" means one that prohibits the use or disclosure of protected health information for any purpose besides the litigation at issue and that requires that all such information be returned to the HIPAA-covered entity (i.e., the psychiatrist) or destroyed when the litigation is finished.

1. Speak with an experienced health care attorney who can advise you. Keep in mind that state law may apply if it is more protective of patient privacy. If your attorney agrees, follow steps 2–4.
2. Speak with your patient and his or her attorney about whether they will provide you with a written authorization to release information and testify. (Again, if you keep "psychotherapy notes" as defined by HIPAA, you must have a specific authorization form.)
3. If the patient's attorney will not provide you with an authorization from the patient, ask the attorney to file a motion to quash or a motion for a qualified protective order. That will lead to a court order from the judge.
4. If this procedure does not work, send a written notice to the attorney who had the subpoena issued. This notice should be tailored to your particular circumstances and may include the following: "In order to release records or testify pursuant to the subpoena which was served on me on [date], I must receive one of the following: a) written, informed authorization from [patient's name] to release the information requested [and specific authorization for release of psychotherapy notes, if applicable]; or b) a court order (qualified to comply with HIPAA) to release the information specified in the subpoena.[2]

## #3: Reporting Duties

As discussed in the previous section, the general rule for psychiatrists is that information learned from the therapeutic relationship should be treated as confidential and not released without patient permission, unless a legally and ethically recognized exception applies. Some of these exceptions have taken the form of legal mandates to "report" certain actions to a designated governmental authority. For example, all states have statutes requiring reports of child abuse.

Additionally, most states have enacted laws that require reports of abuse or neglect of vulnerable adults and/or elderly persons. Some states have also imposed legal requirements on physicians to report certain conditions, such as epilepsy, to the agency overseeing motor vehicle licensing. Others have imposed a broader duty on physicians to report patients diagnosed with a variety of disorders that may impair their driving. If an impaired

---

[2]There may be limits on release of psychotherapy notes as defined by HIPAA; additionally, a qualified protective order must meet all the requirements of the HIPAA Privacy Rule at 45 CFR § 164.512 (e).

driver is not reported in one of the states with such a statute, the physician may be liable for damages to an injured third party.

Most jurisdictions do not have statutes that specifically address the reporting of impaired patients. Some case precedent suggests that psychiatrists may be held liable for failure to warn of the side effects of medication if it could adversely affect driving. It is possible that a court could likewise find liability, under a common-law theory of negligence, for failing to report a patient with alcohol impairment. However, this is an issue regarding which there is little clear-cut precedent. At least the psychiatrist might warn the patient of the danger in drinking and driving, try to enlist the help of family members to curtail driving, and/or convince the patient to voluntarily give up driving or to self-report. Any action taken, or ruled out, should be fully documented.

Many states, through statute or administrative regulation, now require psychiatrists to report medical or mental health colleagues to the appropriate licensure board if such colleagues have engaged in unprofessional conduct. The issue becomes even more complex when the psychiatrist learns of the alleged unprofessional conduct from the patient and the patient wishes to preserve confidentiality. Which duty must the psychiatrist then uphold: the duty to report or the duty to preserve confidentiality? This is a difficult question that must be answered on a case-by-case basis. Psychiatrists are advised to seek both legal and ethical advice when these difficult issues arise. Information may also be sought from the psychiatrist's medical licensure board.

## #4: Recordkeeping

Creating and maintaining accurate records of psychiatric treatment is not an option; it has become the standard of care. At the present time, there is no one standard governing the format of psychiatric records. However, practice settings (e.g., hospitals or agencies) may dictate the types of records that must be maintained. Furthermore, third-party payers, including Medicare and Medicaid, frequently dictate the content of medical records.

How long must records be kept? The new HIPAA Privacy Rule does not address overall clinical record retention but does address retention of records that demonstrate how compliance with the HIPAA Privacy Rule was achieved. Under HIPAA, certain documents (including those relating to use and disclosure of information, as well as the "Notice of Privacy Practices," authorization forms, responses to a patient who wishes to amend his or her record, and the complaint record) must be kept for a minimum of

6 years. However, state law frequently addresses the issue of record retention for medical records. Psychiatrists should check with their state medical licensure boards to determine requirements, if any, in their states. Usually, for outpatient psychiatric records, the required minimum record retention period is not more than 6 or 7 years for adult patients. However, psychiatrists should realize that there is not always a "statute of limitations"[3] for licensure board complaints brought by disgruntled patients. With that in mind, some psychiatrists may wish to keep their records for a longer time period so that they can use the records to demonstrate the care rendered to the patient. Additionally, psychiatrists who treat Medicare and Medicaid patients will generally want to keep their records for at least 10 years, in order to defend against a possible "false claims" action. States frequently require minors' records to be kept for a set period beyond the time when the patient reaches the age of majority.

Psychiatrists may be tempted to add information to the chart after a suicide, homicide, or other adverse event that leads to a malpractice case. Information added after the incident occurs will usually appear to be self-serving. Even worse, some physicians change or destroy certain information in the record after an untoward incident. Such actions can be very damaging to the defendant physician in a subsequent lawsuit.

## #5: The Patient Who Poses a Risk of Harm to Self or Others

Prior to the *Tarasoff* decision in California in the mid-1970s, psychiatrists were rarely found responsible for their patients' acts of violence against a third party (Tarasoff v. Regents of the University of California 1976). The facts leading to this seminal case were as follows: The patient, Prosenjit Poddar, had been a student who was treated by a psychologist at the University of California counseling center. The psychologist became convinced that the patient would try to kill a young woman named Tatiana Tarasoff, so he had the campus police detain Poddar so that civil commitment could be initiated. The police detained him but then released him because they did not believe there was a basis to hold him. The supervising psychiatrist later decided there was no grounds for commitment. The patient terminated treatment and killed Tarasoff.

Tarasoff's parents sued the psychiatrist, the psychologist, and the uni-

---

[3]A statute of limitations is typically an "affirmative defense" to a lawsuit. It does not preclude a patient from filing suit, but the defendant can raise it in an attempt to get the suit dismissed. Although there are state variations, the typical statute of limitations in a medical malpractice action involving an adult patient is 2–3 years.

versity, claiming that they could have taken further action, including warning Tarasoff of the danger posed to her by Poddar. The California Supreme Court agreed and held that after a therapist determines, or pursuant to applicable professional standards should have determined, that a patient poses a risk of violence to a third party, the therapist has a duty to protect the foreseeable victim from that danger (Tarasoff v. Regents 1976). The court explained that the discharge of the duty by the therapist may require one or more steps, depending on the facts. These steps may include warning the intended victim, notifying the police, or taking other reasonable steps according to the particular circumstances.

The *Tarasoff* case led to a series of judicial decisions in numerous states, as well as legislation, recognizing a duty on the part of psychiatrists to warn or protect victims against patient violence. Additionally, many states have enacted statutes that provide immunity to psychiatrists and other mental health professionals if they take certain actions (e.g., warning or notifying the police) in response to a patient's threat to harm a third party.

In addition to liability to third parties as a result of a patient's violence, the number of lawsuits alleging negligence on the part of psychiatrists due to patient suicide or attempted suicide has increased dramatically in the past 30 years. The most common suicide lawsuits involve inpatients, and liability frequently turns on whether policies and procedures were followed, whether reasonable decisions were made concerning discharge and release on passes, and whether there was adequate communication between psychiatrist and staff or psychiatrist and family.

Rather than engage in a lengthy discussion of the case law involving both duty to warn/protect and duty to prevent suicide, I will set forth here some practical pointers for dealing with potentially violent or suicidal patients:

1. *Discuss issues of confidentiality and limits to confidentiality at the outset of treatment.* Although it is advisable to inform patients that you will do everything reasonably necessary to protect confidentiality, it is important to let them know that you may be obligated to breach confidentiality if they pose a risk of harm to themselves or others, or if they engage in other behavior that is reportable by law, such as child or elder abuse. If you are a HIPAA-covered entity, the exceptions to confidentiality should be specified in your "Notice of Privacy Practices."

2. *Be attentive to signs of potential violence or potential harm to self.* In taking an initial history and at other times of major decision-making during treatment, you will want to ask, when it is relevant to do so, about past history of violence, access to weapons, and suicidal or homicidal ideation. When there is cause for concern, it is advisable to make efforts to obtain past treatment records. The outcome in many dangerous-patient

and suicide cases has hinged on whether there was a past history of violence or suicide attempts.

3. *Consult with colleagues and legal counsel when difficult issues arise.* Even if an outcome is less than desirable, you can reduce your risk of liability if you have carefully considered all alternatives and have taken the time to consult with peers and/or legal counsel. In the legal arena, two heads are often better than one. You are held to the "standard of care," which means that you are judged according to what another reasonable psychiatrist would have done under the circumstances. Additionally, a colleague or legal counsel may offer objective alternatives that you may not have considered.

4. *Engage in careful analysis of the situation and take appropriate action.* You should evaluate all options that are pertinent to the particular clinical situation. Have you considered all appropriate options, such as warning the intended victim, notifying the police, hospitalization, and increasing medication? Be especially cautious if a threat against a specific identifiable victim is coupled with a past history of violence; warning is frequently indicated in such circumstances. If you are working with a team in an inpatient setting, is everyone on the team communicating regularly? Have you reviewed recent treatment records created by other members of the treatment team before making important decisions like discharge or release of the patient on pass? If you are supervising nonmedical therapists, have you instructed them to notify you if they become concerned about a patient's potential for suicide or harm to others? Have you exhausted all appeals to the managed care company if continued treatment is denied?

   If the patient is in crisis, it is not typically a good time to consider termination of the psychiatrist-patient relationship. It may be appropriate, in certain cases, to terminate when a patient is in a secure inpatient setting, under the care of another physician.

5. *Make referrals where indicated.* If you are treating a patient with a serious and life-threatening eating disorder, have you considered referrals to a specialist and possibly a cardiologist? If psychological testing is indicated, are you careful to follow up and make sure the patient complies with your recommendation? If you function as a psychiatrist who engages only in medication management, do you ensure that the patient is receiving psychotherapy where indicated? Would a partial hospitalization program help when the needed level of care has moved beyond what you can give?

6. *Document all considerations and actions taken.* Psychiatric records often reflect signs of potential suicide or violence without adequate discussion of what actions were taken to address the potential for harm. It is help-

ful to document the following: patient behavior or statements that are of concern; what your options are; any consultation obtained; what steps you ruled out and why; and what actions you ultimately decided to take and why. For example, if you decided against hospitalization, you should fully document why you decided it was not warranted. If you determined that the patient's statements indicated fantasy as opposed to a realistic threat, you will want to document this in detail. Thorough decision-making, even if somewhat ambiguous, is preferable to creation of a false sense of certainty.

7. *Never alter a record after an adverse outcome.* As discussed earlier, resist the temptation to alter the record after a suicide or violent act by the patient directed to a third party. Experts in analyzing both hand-written and computer records can frequently ascertain that an entry was made after the alleged date of entry. Alteration of records frequently leads to a settlement or judgment against the physician in a malpractice case.

8. *Ensure appropriate follow-up.* Appropriate follow-up may be especially important in an inpatient setting. A patient who appears fine on the date of discharge could decompensate quickly if he or she fails to take medication or doesn't show up for outpatient treatment. Make sure discharge instructions are given, and consider a mechanism whereby someone on staff checks to make sure the patient is following postdischarge instructions.

9. *Familiarize yourself with policies and procedures of any hospitals, agencies, or other institutions where you practice.* Smart legal counsel for the plaintiff will typically obtain copies of relevant policies and procedures. If you do not follow the internal policies of your institution, it may be a great help to the plaintiff's attorney in a malpractice action against you. For example, if you or the staff ignore your facility's procedures for placing a suicidal patient on "maximum observation" or the equivalent status, it may be difficult to defend against a negligence claim.

10. *Keep up to date with changes in ethics and the law.* Psychiatrists may wish to subscribe to publications that will keep them abreast of new case law and statutory changes on the state and federal level. Checking the Web sites of the APA and other physician organizations will help you navigate legal waters without having to go to law school in order to practice medicine.

## #6: Compliance With Medicare/Medicaid and Other Federal Mandates

Psychiatrists new to private practice are entering during an era in which "compliance" with government-imposed duties is expected in many areas.

Many publicized "fraud and abuse" cases have caused psychiatrists to rethink their billing practices, contracting with third-party payers and relationships with employees and independent contractors. In recent years, psychiatrists have faced increased exposure to both civil and criminal penalties for noncompliance with federal and state laws governing fraud and abuse.

The "false claims" provisions of the Social Security Act (§ 1128B(a); 42 USCA § 1320a-7b(a) set forth *criminal* penalties (many of which are felonies) for a variety of actions, including knowingly and willfully making false statements in any application for payment under a federal health care program, including a claim for physician services made while knowing that the person who furnished the services is not a licensed physician. HIPAA broadened the scope of the prohibitions to include knowing and willful fraud against certain *private* plans or contracts affecting commerce (18 USCA § 1347). Furthermore, under the Federal False Claims Act (31 USCA § 3729), substantial *civil* monetary penalties may be imposed on physicians who knowingly submit false claims. However, "knowingly" is defined by the statute to encompass more than acts where a person has actual knowledge; it also includes acts in reckless disregard of the truth or falsity of the information. Any psychiatrist entering private practice should consider hiring staff who are well trained in filling out claims forms so as to comply with the law. Only a well-trained office assistant would know, for example, that a routine waiver of Medicare Part B co-payments could be considered a misstatement of the charge for service and therefore be considered a false claim. A solo practitioner without office staff should make it a priority to learn about the nuances of psychiatric billing and coding. (For further discussion, see Chapter 6 in this volume.)

Another federal law with which psychiatrists should be familiar is the Federal Health Care Program Anti-Kickback Statute. This law makes it a felony for anyone to "knowingly and willfully offer, pay, solicit or receive any remuneration (including any kickback, bribe or rebate) for referring a patient for services covered by Medicare or Medicaid.[4] This statute, along with its "safe harbors" for certain business arrangements, is of utmost importance in negotiating health care contracts. For example, many psychiatrists lease office space to psychologists, social workers, and other nonmedical therapists. It is important to know that, in order to come under a "safe harbor" (to avoid prosecution and exclusion from the Medicare pro-

---

[4]Social Security Act § 1128B(b); 42 USCA § 1320a–7b(b). The scope of the anti-kickback provisions was expanded to a larger group of health plans by HIPAA. Social Security Act § 1128B(f); 42 USCA § 1320a-7b(f).

gram), a lease agreement of this type should have a term of at least 1 year and should be consistent with fair market value, among other requirements. Psychiatrists entering into such agreements should consult with competent health care counsel before any contract is signed.

The physician self-referral law and regulations, commonly referred to as "Stark I and Stark II,"[5] are yet another set of federal mandates affecting psychiatrists. The Stark laws and regulations were enacted to prevent physicians with financial interests in certain entities from referring patients to that entity. Although the Stark I prohibition was limited to physician-owned clinical laboratories and to Medicare services, Stark II extended the referral ban to certain "designated health services" for which Medicare or Medicaid would otherwise pay. These designated health services include clinical laboratory services, physical therapy (including speech pathology), occupational therapy, radiology, radiation therapy services and supplies, durable medical equipment, parenteral and enteral supplies, prosthetics, home health services, outpatient prescription drugs, and inpatient and outpatient hospital services. The regulations are extremely complex but do allow some exceptions, especially where services are provided at fair market value. However, violations can be very costly (up to $15,000 per offending bill or claim and up to $100,000 for certain arrangements or circumvention schemes that do not comport with Stark requirements). Violations can also lead to exclusion from the Medicare and Medicaid programs.

Beyond the Medicare and Medicaid mire, psychiatrists who have a hospital-based practice should also familiarize themselves with EMTALA, the Emergency Medical Treatment and Active Labor Act (1986), the law that was intended to prevent "dumping" of indigent noninsured patients. EMTALA requires that all hospitals participating in Medicare, along with their outpatient clinics, provide an appropriate medical *screening* examination to any person who comes to the hospital seeking emergency services. Furthermore, EMTALA imposes an obligation to *stabilize* any patient determined to have an emergency condition prior to discharge or transfer. Some states have also enacted laws that mirror, or expand upon, the federal requirements.

Although the law targets hospitals, certain penalties may be imposed on physicians who violate the anti-dumping provisions. For example, a physi-

---

[5]Stark I was enacted as part of the Omnibus Budget Reconciliation Act of 1989 (OBRA 89), Pub. L. No. 101-239, 103 Stat. 2106 (1989); Stark II was enacted as part of the Omnibus Budget Reconciliation Act of 1993 (OBRA 93), Pub. L. No. 103-66, 107 Stat. 312 (1993). See also Social Security Act § 1877(g), 42 USCA § 1395nn, and 42 CFR Parts 411 and 424.

cian who is responsible for the screening examination, treatment, or transfer of a patient and who neglects his or her own responsibilities under the law is subject to a penalty of up to $50,000 per violation. Additionally, on-call physicians who fail or refuse to appear within a reasonable time frame are subject to similar penalties. Physicians with gross, flagrant, or repeated violations of EMTALA are subject to exclusion from the Medicare program.

Yet another federal mandate derives from what is now commonly referred to as the "ADA" (Americans With Disabilities Act of 1990). The ADA, which became effective in 1992, requires the provision of appropriate auxiliary aids and services to ensure adequate communication between a physician and a patient with hearing or vision impairments. Although the ADA does not require the use of an interpreter for a deaf or hearing-impaired person in every instance, the key is effective communication. Note-taking, lip reading, or interpretation by a family member may not be considered effective communication when one is engaging in psychotherapy with a patient. Furthermore, a health care professional is not required to provide an interpreter where this would present an "undue burden" on the professional. However, the single factor of interpreter cost exceeding the cost of the medical consultation has not been found by the courts to be an undue burden. Factors that may tilt the determination toward an "undue burden" include the practice's overall income and eligibility for tax credits and the frequency of patient visits requiring an interpreter. Further information on such issues may be obtained from the United States Department of Justice, Civil Rights Division, Public Access Section.[6]

## #7: Managed Care (Minimizing Liability and Reviewing Contracts)

Psychiatrists practicing in the twenty-first century typically participate in some form of managed care. The expansion of HMOs, PPOs, and other varieties in the alphabet soup of managed care has led to an increasing number of legal and risk management concerns for psychiatrists. These

---

[6]The information line at the Department of Justice for issues related to Americans With Disabilities Act compliance and the need for interpreters is 1-800-514-0301. Additionally, some psychiatrists and programs that receive federal financial assistance may have an obligation to provide assistance to patients who do not speak their language. This obligation may not apply to physicians who are merely Medicare Part B recipients. See Title VI Guidelines at http://www.hhs.gov/ocr/lep/revisedlep.html. Accessed July 28, 2004.

concerns range from confidentiality concerns to an increased risk of civil lawsuits to contractual liability.

The HIPAA Privacy Rule does not require providers to obtain patient consent to turn over information to a third party payer as long as the required "Notice of Privacy Practices" is given to the patient. However, the Privacy Rule does permit providers to obtain such consent and, absent an emergency, prior authorization is strongly encouraged by the American Psychiatric Association (2001/2003). Additionally, state law may require advance patient consent or authorization before turning mental health information over to an insurance company or other third party.

Psychiatrists should be aware that managed care companies typically do not have the same accountability that physicians have when clinical decisions are made. The United States Supreme Court issued a long-awaited decision on June 21, 2004, that negated efforts on the part of some states to give patients the right to sue managed care companies for damages where the companies have refused to cover treatment that a physician has deemed medically necessary (Aetna Health Inc v. Davila 2004). In this case, the court ruled that patients'-rights laws of Texas and nine other states[7] are preempted by the federal law commonly known as "ERISA" (Employee Retirement Income Security Act 1974). Unless the United States Congress passes a patients'-rights law, patients' recourse will be limited to suing physicians and related health care entities for malpractice and pursuing administrative remedies for the managed care companies' denial of treatment.

As a practical matter, what can psychiatrists do to lessen their risks in working in a managed care environment? First, it is very important for psychiatrists to discuss with patients the possible limitations on reimbursement. Payment for treatment may be disallowed even if both psychiatrist and patient believe that it is medically indicated.

Second, psychiatrists should be aware that there is a body of legal precedent that suggests that physicians may have a legal duty to appeal adverse utilization review decisions.[8] Appeals procedures are often set forth in a "provider manual," which the psychiatrist should request at the time of contracting. Additionally, some states and certain accrediting bodies for review companies have often promulgated procedural requirements and appeal mechanisms. In making an appeal, the psychiatrist should explain the

---

[7]Arizona, California, Georgia, Maine, New Jersey, North Carolina, Oklahoma, Washington, and West Virginia have enacted comparable laws.

[8] The first in a line of such cases was *Wickline v. State*, 192 Cal. App. 3d 1630, 239 Cal. Rptr. 810 (1986).

necessity for treatment and the possible health risks that would occur if treatment were to be discontinued. The clarity of the clinical records can be crucial in helping the patient obtain necessary treatment. However, it is important not to grossly exaggerate the patient's clinical condition because this could result in the patient's being denied disability, life, or other insurance in the future.

Psychiatrists should be careful not to terminate patient care abruptly if a patient's benefits are discontinued. Termination during a crisis (e.g., with a suicidal patient) often leads to liability for "abandonment" if the patient does attempt or actually accomplish the suicide.

At the time of contracting with managed care entities, it is advisable to seek appropriate consultation. If a psychiatrist is contractually obligated to "indemnify and hold harmless" the managed care company, the psychiatrist is agreeing to take on the liability of the company. The psychiatrist should check with his or her professional liability insurance carrier to ascertain whether coverage may be affected by such assumption of liability by contract. Additionally, because of the financial instability of some managed care companies in recent years, the contractual language should be checked to ensure that the psychiatrist is not obligated to treat patients for long periods of time without payment if the entity becomes insolvent. Psychiatrists may wish to consider the American Medical Association's Model Managed Care Contract, with supplements on many issues including bankruptcy and confidentiality (American Medical Association 2004).

## #8: Collaborative Treatment With Other Mental Health Professionals

In today's managed care environment, treatment responsibilities are often divided; the psychiatrist manages medication while a nonmedical therapist provides the psychotherapy. If the collaborative relationship is good, benefits include possible cost containment, enhanced patient compliance with treatment, and better matching of therapist with patient (Riba et al. 1999). If the split in treatment functions is mismanaged, the patient may be harmed and the potential for liability for the psychiatrist increases.

The psychiatrist engaged in a professional relationship with a nonmedical therapist should first clarify his or her own role: Is the psychiatrist acting as a supervisor (which implies overall responsibility for treatment) or in a collaborative relationship (in which treatment responsibility is shared)? Another alternative may be that the psychiatrist is acting as a consultant, in which case his or her role may be more limited. These roles are defined in great detail by the APA (American Psychiatric Association Guidelines 1980).

There are distinct liability risks inherent in the divided-treatment model. For example, if a patient commits suicide after a session with his or her psychologist, the psychiatrist doing the medication management is also likely to be included in the lawsuit. The plaintiff's lawyer will often used a "shotgun approach" and sue everyone involved in the patient's care. This is frequently referred to as the "sue every deep pocket" phenomenon (Lazarus et al. 1997). Additionally, in many states, a theory of "joint and several liability" applies in malpractice litigation. What this means is that if two or more defendants are determined to have contributed in any amount to the damage suffered by the plaintiff, the injured plaintiff can collect the entire amount from any of the defendants. This could, in certain cases, leave the "less negligent" psychiatrist with the entire judgment.

There are ways in which a psychiatrist can provide good care to the patient while protecting himself or herself at the same time. First, the psychiatrist can discuss the arrangement with the therapist and patient and follow the discussion with an agreement signed by all three parties: the psychiatrist, psychotherapist and patient. (See Appendix 9–A, "Model Collaborative Treatment Relationship Agreement.") The goal of the three-way agreement is to foster good, collaborative communication among the three parties and clarify the roles and responsibilities of each. This agreement may also be drafted to include patient authorization to exchange information between psychiatrist and therapist.

Second, if possible, the psychiatrist should screen therapists with whom he or she agrees to work. The psychiatrist in private practice should check the licensure status and malpractice insurance levels of all therapists with whom he or she is collaborating. The psychiatrist (or group or agency) should require copies of the therapists' professional liability insurance face sheets or policy declarations pages, or request certificates of insurance. These documents should be updated annually.

Third, the psychiatrist should figure out if he or she is willing to take on the risk of a pure "medication management" practice. Many psychiatrists today are treating patients with severe depression and anxiety, who may be suicidal at any time. Common sense and simple math dictate that the psychiatrist who sees 100 or more patients per week for medication management will run a greater malpractice risk than the psychiatrist who sees 35 patients weekly for therapy and medication management combined. In some practice settings (e.g., community health agencies), the psychiatrist has little choice regarding the mix of patients scheduled. Some psychiatrists do negotiate part-time work in these settings so that they can mitigate the risks inherent in dealing with large numbers of patients.

Fourth, when working with nonphysician therapists in a managed care setting, if the therapist refuses to work in a collaborative relationship with the psychiatrist, the psychiatrist should consider notifying the managed care entity. If lack of cooperation continues, the therapist may wish to terminate the contractual arrangement with the managed care company in question.

Fifth, the psychiatrist should always be mindful of clarifying the meaning of his or her signature on any treatment plan or insurance form. For example, a signature on a treatment plan may mean that the psychiatrist reviewed it and approved of the diagnosis and the plan. It does not necessarily mean that he or she saw the patient. The psychiatrist may need to write a qualification such as, "Reviewed and approved by [name]." Likewise, on an insurance or other billing form, the psychiatrist may need to clarify whether he or she performed the services or supervised the therapy by a nonmedical therapist. A useful tool for psychiatrists is the APA's "Guidelines Regarding Psychiatrists' Signatures" (American Psychiatric Association 1989).

## #9: Malpractice Insurance

Professional liability insurance is a major practice-related expense for all physicians in today's litigious society. However, there is more to consider in purchasing a policy than merely the cost of the annual premium. Financial condition of the underwriter, type of policy, claims handling, experience with psychiatric issues, and added value are all important considerations in choosing a policy.

In recent years, many physicians have found themselves without coverage because of financial insolvency of their insurance carriers. Even if the psychiatrist lives in a state with a "guaranty fund," the protection may not be enough to satisfy a major claim. A relatively simple way of protecting the assets of a psychiatric practice is to periodically check the financial stability of one's professional liability insurance companies. A.M. Best, Standard and Poor's, Moody's Investor Services, and Weiss Research, Inc., are all companies that rate insurance companies. If the insurer's rating has been downgraded, the psychiatrist who has been checking the ratings will be in a better position than his or her colleagues to make a change before it's too late.

Another factor in choosing a policy is a basic understanding of the differences among policy types. Two major forms of professional liability insurance in the medical field are policies written on an "occurrence" basis and policies written on a "claims made" basis. For example, if a psychiatrist has an occurrence policy with ABC Company in the year 2005, discontinues coverage in 2006, and is sued in 2007 for a negligent "occurrence" in 2005, the psychiatrist should still be covered in 2007. If a psychiatrist has a "claims made" policy in 2005, discontinues coverage in 2006, and is sued in 2007 for an allegedly negligent act or omission that took place in 2005, he or she will not be covered in 2007 because the claim was not made when the policy was in force. The psychiatrist would, however, be covered if he or she had purchased "tail coverage" when discontinuing the policy.

It is important to note the differences in coverage because premiums are typically much higher in the early years of an occurrence policy. Premiums start out at a lower rate with a claims-made policy but typically escalate in subsequent years. In some markets, an occurrence-type policy may not even be available as an option for psychiatrists because of the potential indefinite exposure for the insurance carrier.

Another consideration is how claims are handled by a particular carrier. For example, is an attorney involved at the outset? Will the insurer assign separate legal counsel if more than one defendant is covered by the same carrier? Will the psychiatrist have any input regarding whether a case should be settled? The latter concern is especially important because medical malpractice settlements and judgments must be reported to the National Practitioner Data Bank (National Practitioner Data Bank 2004).

A psychiatrist may also wish to inquire about the particular experience of the staff in handling psychiatric, as opposed to general medical, claims. A program that insures a large number of psychiatrists will likely be able identify appropriate experts and readily assess the merits of a claim. Likewise, such a program will probably hire attorneys with experience in mental health matters.

One more factor in purchasing a policy is the "value added" part of the insurance package. Some programs provide risk management advice to insureds at no extra cost; others do not. Some insurance policies cover defense costs to defend against complaints before state licensure boards and other administrative bodies; others do not. The wise purchaser of a malpractice policy will find out exactly what benefits are included as part of the policy.

## #10: e-Psychiatry

*Telemedicine, telehealth, e-psychiatry, computerized medical record (CMR)*, and *electronic health record (EHR)* are just some of the myriad high-tech words that have inundated the lexicon of the modern psychiatrist. Although use of computers, facsimile machines, and e-mail can facilitate communication, they can also create legal minefields for the practicing psychiatrist. The following are some of the important issues for psychiatrists to consider in this new era of medical practice.

First, psychiatrists considering Internet practice should be aware that many states' licensure boards interpret their laws as requiring physicians to be licensed where the patient is located. The American Telemedicine Association has argued for the end of individual state licensure for telemedicine activities (American Telemedicine Association 2004). The Federation of State Medical Boards has drafted a model telemedicine licensure act that would regulate telemedicine practice across state lines but it has not been adopted as proponents had hoped. Some states have adopted limited telemedicine license laws but many still require full licensure for telemedicine practice. Additionally, psychiatrists should check with their liability insurance carriers to determine if they have coverage for telemedicine activities, especially if conducted outside of the psychiatrists' home states.

Second, psychiatrists should be careful to develop procedures for dealing with e-mail and computerized records. (See earlier discussion of HIPAA.) For example, confidential information should generally not be sent via e-mail to psychiatric patients, especially where the e-mail might be read by another member of the patient's household or workplace. Faxes should be sent, with great care, only to a particular intended person who is waiting to receive the fax, and only with patient authorization. Computers with confidential information should not be passed on to another owner or "dumped" without deleting the sensitive information stored on the hard drive.

Third, psychiatrists should keep abreast of new ethical guidelines and laws regarding computerized records and electronic exchange of confidential information. Since the advent of HIPAA, the National Committee for Vital and Health Statistics (NCVHS) has been working to establish standards for information and terminology regarding electronic health records. Widespread changes in creation and maintenance of medical records will certainly affect psychiatric practice in the future.

## ■ CONCLUSION

Psychiatrists today are subject to a much greater level of regulation and oversight of their practices than their counterparts of 20 or more years ago. However, with reasonable diligence, proper documentation, involvement in professional associations, and appropriate consultation with colleagues and other professionals, the typical psychiatrist will be able to conduct his or her practice with a high degree of success and satisfaction. Education does not end with medical school; it is a lifelong process for the competent psychiatrist.

# ▮ REFERENCES

Aetna Health Inc v Davila, 124 S Ct 2488 (2004)

American Medical Association: Model Managed Care Contract and supplements. Available at: http://www.ama-assn.org/ama/pub/category/9559.html. Accessed July 28, 2004.

American Psychiatric Association: Guidelines for psychiatrists in consultative, supervisory, or collaborative relationships with nonmedical therapists. Am J Psychiatry 127:1489–1491, 1980

American Psychiatric Association: Guidelines regarding psychiatrists' signatures. APA Document Reference No. 890002, 1989. [See also Sederer LI, Ellison JM, Keyes C: Guidelines for Prescribing Psychiatrists in Consultative, Collaborative, and Supervisory Relationships. Psychiatr Serv 49:1197–2002, 1998]

American Psychiatric Association: Principles of Medical Ethics with Annotations Especially Applicable to Psychiatry, Sec. 4, 2 (2001 edition, including 2003 amendments)

American Psychiatric Association: Member's Corner. HIPAA Education Packet. Available at: http://www.psych.org/members/hipaa/hipaa_packet.cfm. Accessed August 25, 2004.

American Telemedicine Association. Available at: http://www.atmeda.org. Accessed August 30, 2004.

Americans with Disabilities Act of 1990, 42 USCA § 12101 et seq

Centers for Medicare and Medicaid Services ("CMS"): Decision-making tool to clarify "covered entity" status under HIPAA. Available at: http://www.cms.hhs.gov/hipaa/hipaa2/support/tools/decisionsupport/default.asp. Accessed July 28, 2004.

Emergency Medical Treatment and Active Labor Act ("EMTALA"). 42 USCA § 1395dd (Section 1867 of the Social Security Act)

Employee Retirement Income Security Act of 1974, Pub. L. No. 93-406, 88 Stat. 829

Health Privacy Project. Available at: http://www.healthprivacy.org. Accessed August 25, 2004.

Jaffee v Redmond, 518 US 1 (1996)

Lazarus J, Macbeth J, Wheeler N: Divided treatment in the managed care arena: legal and ethical risks. Psychiatric Practice and Managed Care, March-April 1997

National Practitioner Data Bank: Practitioner's Guide to the Databanks. Available at: http://npdb-hipdb.com. Accessed July 28, 2004.

Office for Civil Rights, U.S. Department of Health and Human Services: Sample Business Associate Contract Provisions. August 2002. Available at: http://www.hhs.gov/ocr/hipaa/contractprov.html. Accessed August 25, 2004.

Office for Civil Rights, U.S. Department of Health and Human Services. Available at: http://www.hhs.gov/ocr/hipaa. Accessed August 25, 2004.

Riba MB, Balon R (eds): Psychopharmacology and Psychotherapy. Washington, DC, American Psychiatric Press, 1999

Tarasoff v Regents of the University of California, 17 Cal. 3d 425, 551 P.2d 334 (1976)

Workgroup for Electronic Data Interchange 2004. Available at: http://snip.wedi.org. Accessed July 28, 2004.

## APPENDIX 9–A

# Model Collaborative Treatment Relationship Agreement

[Patient's Name] ("Patient") has requested that [Psychiatrist's Name] ("Psychiatrist") manage his/her psychiatric medications while he/she concurrently sees [Psychotherapist's Name] ("Therapist") for psychotherapy. This agreement will help facilitate Patient's treatment by clarifying the respective roles and modes of communication of Psychiatrist and Therapist and ensuring that Patient understands them.

Since Therapist will typically be in more frequent contact with Patient, Therapist (or the psychotherapist covering for him/her) will be available at all times to Patient for emergency intervention and will respond within a reasonable period of time. Patient understands that he/she is to contact the Therapist initially in any crisis or situation where hospitalization or some other urgent, non-medication-related care may be necessary. Therapist will contact Psychiatrist as needed in such emergencies. Patient, however, will initially contact Psychiatrist only in the case of emergencies involving medication side effects or in the event that he/she is unable to reach Therapist (or the psychotherapist covering for him/her).

Moreover, since good communication between providers is important for the success of a collaborative relationship such as this, Psychiatrist and Therapist agree to return each other's phone calls promptly, and to inform each other in a timely manner if Patient fails to keep appointments or otherwise comply with treatment recommendations. In the event that Patient terminates with Psychiatrist or Therapist, that provider shall promptly advise the patient to make an appointment with the other provider in order to review his/her overall treatment plan.

This treatment relationship is collaborative. Patient understands that there is no supervisory or agency relationship between Psychiatrist and Therapist. Each provider practices independently and is free to accept or reject the advice or recommendations made by the other provider. Neither provider has any control over the manner and means of the services performed by the other provider. Each provider will bill patient for his/her services separately.

Psychiatrist, Psychotherapist, and Patient have each read this agreement and understand and assent to its terms.

| | |
|---|---|
| _____ | _____ |
| [Psychiatrist] | [Date] |
| _____ | _____ |
| [Psychotherapist] | [Date] |
| _____ | _____ |
| [Patient] | [Date] |

---

_Note._ This agreement is intended to guide the psychiatrist who is in a nonsupervisory relationship with a therapist who is not a physician.

_Source._ Reprinted, with minor changes, from J. E. Macbeth, A. M. Wheeler, J. W. Sither, et al., _Legal and Risk Management Issues in the Practice of Psychiatry_ (Washington, DC, American Psychiatric Press, 1994, p. 44). Used with the permission of American Psychiatric Publishing, Inc., and Psychiatrists' Purchasing Group, Inc.

# 10 ETHICS IN PRIVATE PRACTICE

*Jeremy A. Lazarus, M.D.*

$B$y the time you've made the decision to enter private practice, you will ideally have had a good grounding in medical ethics, and especially in ethics for psychiatrists. These subjects can be researched in more detail in several excellent publications. From the perspective of organized medicine, the AMA's *Code of Medical Ethics and Current Opinions* of the Council on Ethical and Judicial Affairs (American Medical Association [AMA] 2004) is a good start. For organized psychiatry's perspective, the APA's *Principles of Medical Ethics With Annotations Especially Applicable to Psychiatry* (American Psychiatric Association [APA] 2001/2003) is the place to look. For the recently trained, in a book entitled *Ethics in Mental Health* (Roberts and Dyer 2004) you will find very good and comprehensive discussions about a variety of topics in ethics. The focus of this chapter, however, will be on many of the common ethical situations and conflicts that arise in private practice. The general areas for discussion are the following:

- Confidentiality
- Informed consent
- Beneficence
- Boundaries
- Dealing with industry
- Personal education

- Health care ethics
- Collaboration with others
- Money and ethics

# ∎ CONFIDENTIALITY

Psychiatrists, perhaps more than any other physicians, are consistently trained to respect confidentiality, even beyond the extent that might be provided in the law. It's necessary to be able to assure patients that, with rare exceptions, what they tell you in the confines of your office is between you and them alone. This is particularly true for their clinical treatment but may extend even to their identifying information for billing or other purposes. Yet issues can arise in private practice for which the rules don't always seem to fit. Let me give you a few case vignettes with some discussion on how best to handle these situations:

### Case Vignette 1

You and your wife are at a musical show and one of your patients walks up to you and says hello. Your wife does not know this patient, and he doesn't introduce himself to your wife. After a few pleasant words, your patient bids you adieu. Your wife asks you who that person was. How should you handle this situation?

Discussion. Since your patient didn't introduce himself, it would not be appropriate to tell your wife the patient's name, because this would be a breach of confidentiality. It also would not be appropriate you tell your wife that he was a patient, for the same reasons. You might respond that it's someone you've met elsewhere, not respond at all, or tell your wife you're not able to respond. Over time your wife will learn that these responses may indicate that the person was a patient and will not press for more information. It is surprising how often you will meet your patients or former patients in your social life. It's best to be prepared for this inevitable occurrence and know how you will respond. Of course, if your patient introduces himself to your wife, it's quite all right to introduce your wife. But unless your patient reveals something about your relationship with him, you should refrain from saying more.

### Case Vignette 2

You receive a call from the adult child of one of your patients, who leaves a message on your answering machine that there is important information she would like you to know about your patient. You have not previously received permission to talk to this person. What should you do?

**Discussion.** To adhere strictly to confidentiality requirements, it would probably be best not to return the call to your patient's child until you receive permission from your patient to do so. However, what often works well is to return the call, indicating clearly that you cannot discuss anything about any of your patients without their consent. You might say that you would be willing to listen to whatever the person wants to tell you without any response from you whatsoever. You would also indicate that anything you may hear about a patient from interested others will be shared with the patient. Although this may be frustrating to some who call, this type of response is often met with acceptance, and you may indeed hear information that will be crucial in your care of a patient. It's important to tell your patient about the call and the information that was transmitted and to ask whether the patient wishes you to respond in any other way or get permission for further contact with the patient's child. There will be some situations where the patient will refuse to allow any contact, but others where the patient welcomes family interaction. If you play it safe and do not return the call (unless, of course, there is some evidence of a life-threatening emergency), you are also ethically correct. Good judgment and knowing your patients will also allow you to choose which path to follow.

### Case Vignette 3

Your patient is a famous and well-respected entertainer in your city. You are at a cocktail party where your friends begin an animated conversation about her and ask your opinion about her latest performance. What should you do?

**Discussion.** First, make sure there is nothing in what you say or in how you respond that would indicate that you know her outside of her public persona. Feel free to comment on her performance if you have an opinion, or steer clear by indicating lack of knowledge. It's important not to betray your professional relationship by anything you do. This may take a bit of acting on your part, but it's crucial if we are to be able to treat patients who are well known to the public.

## ▌ INFORMED CONSENT

Informed consent has taken on a larger role as psychiatrists and other physicians try to avoid risk in their practices. However, there is at least one situation that often occurs in which psychiatrists in private practice may err by not obtaining such consent:

### Case Vignette 1

In your practice, you see patients through a psychiatric carveout that requires you to have a personal interaction with a case manager after 10 outpatient visits. The case manager calls you and requests that you discuss various nonsensitive areas of the patient's treatment, such as current medications, response to treatment, diagnosis, and prognosis. The patient has signed a consent form with the carveout company that allows you to share this information. What should you do?

Discussion. Although from a legal point of view your patient has granted informed consent, you should not presume that this exists from an ethical point of view. The patient may not have understood the meaning of the releases signed, may or may not wish you to share information, and may want to contribute to the discussion. The best ethical course for you to follow is to wait until you have discussed the case manager's request with your patient and have reconfirmed the informed consent. It also is entirely reasonable to ask the patient if he or she would like to be in the room during the call so as to hear exactly what you are saying. Often patients prefer not to do that, but offering the option indicates your respect for the patient's opinions and for confidentiality. On rare occasions a patient might not wish you to discuss his or her treatment with a case manager, and you would need to comply with that instruction. Of course, that might preclude the patient's using the insurance benefit.

## ∎ BENEFICENCE

The ethics of the APA and the AMA clearly spell out that a physician's primary obligation is to the patient first and then to self and society. Yet some situations arise in which the obligation to put the patient first may be tested and ethical conflicts may arise. Here is an example:

### Case Vignette 1

You are treating a patient with severe borderline personality traits who has begun waiting at your home, talking to your family, and calling you on frequent occasions at home and at the office. Because this patient has had violent tendencies in the past, you are concerned about the safety of yourself and your family. What should you do?

Discussion. Although your primary responsibility is to your patient, you are also responsible to yourself and your family. If you are unable to establish boundaries that the patient respects, you may need to terminate your care of this patient. Setting appropriate boundaries may also benefit the patient, and this can be discussed as an issue in your treatment. In this example, the best treatment has ethical ramifications that need to be taken into consideration. In some ways, the private setting may not be the best site to treat certain difficult patients. If that is the case, it is ethical to refer such patients to the best treatment facility.

# ▌ BOUNDARIES

It is very clear in the *Annotations* of the APA (American Psychiatric Association 2001/2003) that sexual relationships with current or former patients are unethical. The ethical position of the AMA is less strict regarding former patients, but all physicians are well advised that when it comes to finding sexual partners, it's best to look elsewhere than to current or former patients. Yet psychiatrists and other physicians continue to place their patients and themselves at risk by finding themselves "falling in love" with patients and not realizing that it's unethical (as well as often illegal and against state medical practice regulations). They also find numerous rationalizations for why their particular case is an exception.

More complex are the other boundary issues, whether sharply defined as boundary violations or ranked as problems on a scale of 1 to 10. What you need to keep in mind is the extent to which any boundary issue causes harm to a patient. What may seem like a minor slip in professional boundaries for one patient may turn out to be significant and quite harmful for another patient—especially one who has a history of being traumatized by significant others. Here are some examples:

### Case Vignette 1

You have been seeing a middle-aged adult patient for more than 10 years for medication management of her bipolar disorder. Her condition has been stable, and she sees you once every 3 months for assessment of her medications and follow-up on her life situation. You are not engaged in any ongoing insight-oriented psychotherapy with her. One day the patient asks if you would consider seeing her 23-year-old daughter, who is beginning to have some depressive and hypomanic episodes. What should you do?

**Discussion.** There is no specific ethical prohibition against seeing members of the same family. What needs consideration is the effect, positive or negative, this will have on your existing patient; whether there are any conflicts between mother and daughter that might interfere with your objectivity; and whether the daughter will feel she can fully trust you. One possible course if you're uncertain is to agree to see the daughter in consultation only and to determine at that time whether there will be any therapeutic problems. If problems seem likely to arise, you can refer the daughter to another psychiatrist for ongoing treatment.

Over the course of many years, private practice psychiatrists may develop a family practice of psychiatry in which they see multiple members of the same family. This may be a necessity in rural areas where there are few practicing psychiatrists. It's important to remember that the ethical imperative is to do what is in the best interest of the patient, and potential harm to your original patient should be the first consideration.

### Case Vignette 2

Some friends invite you and a guest to a small dinner party. They indicate that there will be several people there whom you are not familiar with. In the course of the conversation you ask your friends who the individuals are and find out that one of those invited is a patient that you've been seeing in individual psychotherapy for 2 years. What should you do?

Discussion. In this situation the best course of action is to graciously decline the invitation. A small setting such as this may make the patient uncomfortable and may also make you uncomfortable. The possibilities for confidentiality breaches are high. This is less of a problem at a large social gathering at which one of your patients is in attendance, although similar issues may come up. The best approach is to have a good feel for who might be at the smaller social events and avoid those at which you're likely to encounter a patient.

## ▮ DEALING WITH INDUSTRY

The main intersection of psychiatry with industry is with the pharmaceutical companies who provide educational opportunities, medication information, and other resources that can be of benefit to you and your patients. The ethical problems that can arise involve gifts or gift equivalents that may influence your prescribing behavior. This issue is comprehensively discussed in the AMA's *Code of Medical Ethics* under "Gifts to Physicians from Industry." Although many physicians don't believe that a fancy dinner or gift will unduly influence them, there is a body of evidence to suggest that these marketing efforts do indeed influence the prescribing of the company's product. It's very important to provide the best and most scientifically based care that you can, and so caution is urged when accepting anything from pharmaceutical companies. There are also many continuing medical education (CME) activities at which no marketing occurs, and attending these may serve better to benefit you and your patients than receiving product information at a sponsored event. On the other hand, some physicians use the medication samples they receive to try to help indigent patients, and most pharmaceutical companies do provide free medications on request for patients who are unable to afford them.

Nevertheless, there are some cautions to raise about the intersection between these companies and you in a private practice. In a private office, you may have only yourself or perhaps a single staff member between you and a pharmaceutical representative. It's very important to establish guidelines on how you wish to interact with these representatives. You can choose no interaction, meetings by appointment only, or regular meetings. The representatives are barred from offering any significant gifts, but they do bring in small amounts of food to staff or brochures that they may request be handed out or placed in the waiting room. Restricting literature that bears the name of only one company is a good way to keep your office from getting cluttered and looking like an advertising opportunity for the companies. Many patients do appreciate educational materials, though, and these can be obtained from the APA, the National Institute of Mental Health, and other not-for-profit agencies.

## ▌ PERSONAL EDUCATION

One very important ethical duty is to keep up your professional education so that you continue to practice in a competent manner. We all have the obligation to do this. Taking courses, getting supervision or consultation, and doing your own teaching can serve the patients you see and keep you connected with emerging scientific information. Board certification and recertification is another way of demonstrating your commitment to the quality of care you provide, and often this is a requirement for participation in physician networks. You can gain access to excellent courses through the APA, your state district APA branch, numerous commercial educational entities, and your local state and county medical societies. Many states require a certain number of CME hours for relicensure, so why not take CME activities that will have an impact on your practice? On occasion, patients will ask whether you participate in these activities, and certainly the question will be asked if you do any forensic or consultation work.

## ▌ HEALTH CARE ETHICS

Although your focus in private practice will be on the care of your patients, you'll find that a good appreciation for health care ethics in general will serve you and your patients well. The ethical issues that most affect your patients will be the lingering (though diminishing) effects of stigma against the mentally ill; ongoing attempts to achieve full nondiscriminatory coverage for mental illness treatment; and the need to protect the safety of our patients by containing expansion of prescriptive authority by those who have not had appropriate medical training. Unfortunately, on the broader front of health care ethics, more than 45 million people in our country are uninsured, there are disparities in treatment for minorities, and there still is much to do to improve the quality and safety of the care that we render. So, you might ask, how does all of this affect ethics for me in my private practice? Let me give a couple of examples:

### Case Vignette 1

You become aware that in your state there is a bill before the legislature to provide nondiscriminatory mental health services to the citizens of your state. You would like to be a strong advocate for this legislation, but you don't know how you can properly do this with your own patients. What can you do?

Discussion. The AMA's opinions on this issue indicate that advocacy with patients outside of the clinical encounter is permissible. However, opinions rendered by the APA Ethics Committee have tended to be more conservative, suggesting that engaging in activities involving patients but not related to the treatment goals is at the very least discouraged. This position is grounded in concerns about the effects of transference and about undue influence on vulnerable patients. There are a number of ways to deal with this dilemma. One is to become involved with the legislative process through your APA district branch and participate in public education about the legislation. Some psychiatrists provide information in their waiting rooms for public education, and if you think information on an issue such as this will not adversely affect the treatment of your patients, there is no specific ethical prohibition to providing it. It becomes a bit trickier if you initiate a discussion with your patients, and care must be taken to ensure that you are not unduly influencing them. If patients ask you about information in your waiting room, it is appropriate to provide factual information about how the new legislation may affect their own insurance benefits or those of others. Remember that your primary obligation is to your patients and you would not want to adversely affect their treatment. Consultation with your APA district branch ethics committee regarding ethical standards in the community may help you resolve this dilemma.

## Case Vignette 2

One of the patients you serve has insurance coverage through a carveout behavioral health company that performs utilization review on your patient. At one point in treatment, the utilization reviewer denies further coverage for the psychotherapy component of the treatment you are providing and indicates that she will only authorize coverage for medication management. You strongly feel that the best treatment for your patient is a combination of psychotherapy and medication management, yet you don't want to get into a conflict with the carveout company. What should you do?

Discussion.  Your primary obligation is to your patient and to be your patient's advocate. In that context, the ethical course for you to follow is to appeal the denial of psychotherapy services through the entire chain of appeal mechanisms available in that company and to inform your patient of your action. You have an ethical obligation to advocate for necessary treatment, and indeed there is also a legal obligation to advocate for necessary services that has been tested in the courts.

## Case Vignette 3

As an active member of your county and state medical society, you have advocated for a particular type of health care reform proposal that is not supported enthusiastically by the public. As part of your participation, you are asked to have your name attached to an ad that will be running in your local newspaper. You wonder how this will affect your relationship with your patients.

Discussion.  Being a psychiatrist does not mean that you can't engage in activities that benefit the public. Indeed, we have a duty to improve health care for the community. There is wide latitude in how we can do that, ranging from contributing funds to a campaign to being actively involved in promoting the campaign. With each individual patient, it is important to determine whether the patient's knowledge about your other professional activities will adversely affect treatment. Discussion with a supervisor or with colleagues will help guide you to the right solution.

# ▌ COLLABORATION WITH OTHERS

Psychiatrists in any type of practice have an ethical obligation to work collaboratively with others who also care for their patients. On the other hand, there is no ethical obligation to work collaboratively with another health care professional you do not deem to be competent. In private practice, the most likely collaborative treatment will be with other physicians who also care for your patients for their other medical needs. A good, secure, and confidential form of communication will ensure that all physicians treating the patient are up to date on the course of all illnesses, medications administered, and progress in treatment. It is rare for a patient to refuse permission for such collaboration, and it is also highly unusual for other treating physicians to have a significant interest in highly personal information about your patient. For guidance on how to work with primary care physicians, see Chapter 8 of this volume.

Psychiatrists also often work collaboratively with other mental health professionals. This subject is covered in detail in *Psychopharmacology and Psychotherapy: A Collaborative Approach* (Riba and Balon 1999) and in my chapter on ethics in that same book (Lazarus 1999). A number of potentially thorny issues arise in collaborative relationships. With the advent of managed care, it is likely that psychiatrists are taking the role of medication manager while other mental health professionals are providing psychotherapy. This often occurs without the psychiatrist's having a previous working relationship with the other mental health professional. The ethical necessities of collaborating on patient care, being sensitive to personal information, ensuring that others treating the patient are competent to do so, and managing triangulated relationships with the managed care company or behavioral care carveout can produce unpleasant ethical dilemmas. Here are some examples:

### Case Vignette 1

You have agreed to provide medication management services to patients who are referred by a behavioral health carveout, and you understand that patients referred to you may also be seeing another mental health professional for psychotherapy concurrently. You learn from one of your patients that the psychotherapist is providing unnecessary or possibly inappropriate services. What should you do?

Discussion. Because your primary ethical obligation is to the patient, you should first express your concerns to your patient and make sure you have permission to discuss her treatment with the psychotherapist. You should then discuss your concerns with the psychotherapist and determine whether indeed your concerns are justified. If you determine that your concerns are valid, then you should request that the psychotherapist alter the treatment. If that is accepted, then you should continue to monitor that treatment. If it is not accepted, then you can discuss the case with the behavioral health carveout case manager. If you get no satisfaction from that approach, then you can ethically decide to withdraw from the care of that patient. The best outcome in these situations is to try to resolve the dilemma in the interest of the patient. If indeed something untoward is going on in the other treatment and you fail to act, you may be subject to ethical, legal, and possibly licensure risks.

### Case Vignette 2

For a number of your patients, you are working in collaborative treatment with a psychologist whom you greatly respect. The psychologist has become very familiar with your protocols for prescribing medications and asks you if he can make recommendations to the patients, based on written protocols that you will provide, to alter medications for patients you are both treating. How should you respond?

Discussion. It would be unethical and illegal to delegate any medical authority to a non–medically trained individual, especially if it is not within the scope of his own practice. To do so would put your patients and yourself at potential risk. If the other mental health professional were licensed under the scope of his practice to perform these duties, then you would need to decide whether you thought it was safe to have such a treatment relationship. It would not be illegal under those circumstances, but you would still be under no obligation to agree if you thought there was a safety or quality issue.

## ▮ MONEY AND ETHICS

Private practice holds out the opportunity to build a practice on sound business and professional principles and also to earn a decent income. However, it's important not to let the quest for income outweigh your professional obligations. Hence the reminder about dealing cautiously with the pharmaceutical and other industries and doing only what does not come at a cost to your patients, either monetarily or in their treatment. There are no specific prohibitions on the fees you set, although there are some guidelines you can refer to in AMA and APA publications. If your fees turn out to be on the extraordinarily high side in your community, then you may be setting up a situation in which, at the very least, you may undergo some ethical scrutiny from your peers. Make sure that your fees appear fair to you and to your patients and that they reflect the time and expertise that you bring to the patient/physician encounter. Make sure that your fees and issues related to money are clearly articulated and agreed upon by your patients. Issues about fees are often grist for the mill, so to speak, in therapy. However, if your business relationship with the patient is unclear, there is a potential for misunderstandings that can adversely affect your treatment relationship. You certainly have a right to expect to be paid for the services you provide, and to be paid in a timely manner. If you choose to make any deviations from your usual processes for billing or fee collection, make sure that you have a good treatment rationale for the deviation.

The current practice environment may provide financial incentives to see larger numbers of patients for shorter periods of time. These financial incentives may influence the intensity and frequency of services that you provide to individual patients. Try to balance your income needs with a soundly based justification for the type of treatment that you provide and don't be seduced into having a "factory-based" outlook on private practice. It's important to realize that there are realistic limits on the income that can be achieved in private practice and not to aspire to the potential income of our procedurally based medical colleagues. Although you can supplement your income with higher-paying services, as noted in Chapter 1 of this volume, there are limits here also. Unless you become a superstar in a specialized area, your income will change only with the numbers of patients seen and the degree to which you can increase your fees to offset the increase in your expenses.

## ∎ CONCLUSION

Although private practice may be an oasis of autonomy, it is not without external oversight in the form of ethics committees, grievance committees of medical societies, and your medical licensing board. For the most part, however, you'll need to be guided by your own conscience and your understanding of both psychiatric and medical ethics. It's not good enough nowadays to say that you were unaware of the ethical positions of your profession. To maintain good working relationships with your patients, your medical colleagues, and the public, and to maintain the integrity of our profession, it will be incumbent on you in private practice to uphold the highest ethical standards. It's likely that it will also help you sleep well at night and be proud of what you're doing.

## ∎ REFERENCES

American Medical Association: Code of Medical Ethics, Current Opinions. Chicago, IL, American Medical Association, 2004

American Psychiatric Association: The Principles of Medical Ethics With Annotations Especially Applicable to Psychiatry (including November 2003 amendments). 2001/2003. Available at: http://www.psych.org/psych_pract/ethics/ethics.cfm.

Lazarus JA: Ethical issues in divided or collaborative treatment, in Psychopharmacology and Psychotherapy: A Collaborative Approach. Edited by Riba M, Balon R. Washington, DC, American Psychiatric Press, 1999, pp 159–177

Riba M, Balon R (eds): Psychopharmacology and Psychotherapy: A Collaborative Approach. Washington, DC, American Psychiatric Press, 1999

Roberts L, Dyer A: Ethics in Mental Health Care. Washington, DC, American Psychiatric Publishing, 2004

# INDEX

*Page numbers printed in **boldface** type refer to tables, figures, or appendices.*